Lean and Hard

The Body You've Always Wanted in Just 24 Workouts

MACKIE SHILSTONE

John Wiley & Sons, Inc.

Published by John Wiley & Sons, Inc., Hoboken, New Jersey
Published simultaneously in Canada

Design and composition by Navta Associates, Inc.

The information contained in this book is not intended to serve as a replacement for professional medical advice. Any use of the information in this book is at the reader's discretion. The author and the publisher specifically disclaim any and all liability arising directly or indirectly from the use or application of any information contained in this book. A health care professional should be consulted regarding your specific situation.

For general information about our other products and services, please contact our Customer Care Department within the United States at (800) 762-2974, outside the United States at (317) 572-3993 or fax (317) 572-4002.

Wiley also publishes its books in a variety of electronic formats. Some content that appears in print may not be available in electronic books. For more information about Wiley products, visit our web site at www.wiley.com.

Library of Congress Cataloging-in-Publication Data:
Shilstone, Mackie.
 Lean and hard : the body you've always wanted in just 24 workouts / Mackie Shilstone.
  p. cm.
 Includes bibliographical references and index.
 ISBN 978-0-470-03763-8 (cloth)
 1. Physical fitness. 2. Exercise. 3. Muscle strength. I. Title.
 RA781.S552 2007
 613.7'1—dc22
                                                                2006016188

Printed in the United States of America

10 9 8 7 6 5 4 3 2 1

I dedicate this book to my wife, Sandy; my sons, Scott and Spencer; and to all the athletes who gave me the opportunity to touch their lives in a positive way and for the great life experiences we have had along the way. It continues to be a great ride.

Contents

PART FOUR
Your Daily Muscle-Building Guide

      Resources   271

      Index   273

Acknowledgments

I would like to give my heartfelt thanks to the following people for their invaluable help with this book.

My wife loving wife, Sandy, and my sons, Scott and Spencer, for their patience, understanding, and continued loving support in helping me create my fifth book.

Bonnie Solow, my literary agent, who works hard to help my books find an audience so that they can help others and who continues to believe in all I do.

My friend and collaborator, Joy Parker, who over the years has continued to give me her personal insights and to translate my sometimes complex ideas into easy-to-understand prose.

Tom Miller, my editor at John Wiley & Sons, who understands the value of my work and enables it to reach thousands of readers who can most benefit from it.

Jim Flarity, Ph.D., for his diligence in supervising the original twenty candidates in our pilot research program upon which this book is based.

The Louisiana State University Healthcare Network for agreeing to allow us to perform the pilot research program at its facility.

Vince Morelli, M.D., affiliated with the Louisiana State University Family Medicine and Sports Medicine departments, for his willingness to review the manuscript for the accuracy of the medical and physiological data.

James Tebbe, M.D., medical director of Elmwood Fitness Center, and affiliated with the Ochsner Health System's Department of Family Medicine, for his review of the manuscript and his writing of the medical clearance guidelines, as well as his setting up of the supplement usage criteria.

Tavis Piattoly, M.S., R.D., L.D.N., for updating the nutrition and supplement sections of this book and for assisting in the development of the meal plans.

My assistant, Michelle Bordelon, who keeps my program on target so I can focus on my objectives.

Judy Johnson for scanning Bob Anderson's stretching graphics.

Bob and Jean Anderson for allowing me to use parts of their highly regarded stretching program from their book *Stretching* (Shelter Publications, Inc., 2000).

John Williams for sharing his extensive research on supplements for high-performance exercise.

Patrick McCausland for his continued support of my fitness and nutrition projects.

Amerifit, Inc., the source of funding for the original research program upon which this book is based.

Marty Herman, the former president of Amerifit, who had the vision to see the value of the original research program.

The original twenty participants in the pilot program for their diligence and willingness to go the distance with the exercise and nutrition in this program, enabling them to undergo a dramatic physique transformation.

Toby Armstrong, for taking the excellent exercise photographs in this book.

Simonne St. Pe and Mack Chuilli for agreeing to be models for the weight training exercises in this book.

Our copy editor, Faren Bachelis, and our proofreader, Sibylle Kazeroid.

Introduction

They Said It Couldn't Be Done

In 1982, I was contacted by a man named Don Hubbard to develop a nutrition and exercise program for him and his wife, Rose. He was so impressed with the results that he asked me to take on a very special client. Hubbard was one of the principal investors in Michael Spinks, who had won the Olympic gold medal as a middleweight boxer in 1976. Spinks was considered the best light heavyweight boxer in the world and owned two out of three belts in his division.

This was a great opportunity for me. In 1975, I was volunteering as a strength and conditioning coach at Tulane University. In 1982, Spinks became my first pro athlete.

From 1982 to 1985, I became what Hubbard referred to as Spinks's secret weapon. Rather than use what I considered archaic training principles that weren't serving Spinks, I taught him how to better manage his strength, increase his speed and stamina, and perfect his technique. Under my guidance, Spinks went on to become the undisputed world light heavyweight champion, defeating fighter Dwight Braxton, who held the third belt in his division.

Spinks had an even bigger dream: he wanted to increase his strength and lean muscle weight so that he could qualify to fight in the heavyweight category. He would then be able to fight Larry Holmes, the undisputed heavyweight champion of the world. Holmes was a large, fast, and powerful legend, with forty-eight straight wins and every belt in boxing—and this was when opponents fought fifteen rounds instead of the twelve that they fight now.

For thirty years, light heavyweight boxers had been trying to move up and defeat a heavyweight title holder, but it had never been done. While these men had achieved the mandatory weight to challenge the larger men, they had all been defeated. The conventional boxing wisdom of the time was "A good big man will always beat a good little man."

I believed otherwise. As a young man, my goal had been to be a walk-on receiver for a major college football team. At 5' 9" I was the smallest guy at the Tulane University tryouts. Yet I persevered, learning everything I could about high-intensity exercise and performance nutrition, and developed the attitude "Never give up." I became the smallest guy on the team and the smallest college football player in the country, but I won my varsity letter.

Building lean muscle and superior athletic performance in others became my specialty, and I had the knowledge and experience to help Spinks get where he wanted to go.

The Spinks/Holmes fight was set for September 21, 1985. To get Spinks ready for the fight of his life, I worked with him intensively for eight weeks, employing the same basic strategy that I offer readers in this book: high-performance nutrition, performance supplementation, and high-intensity interval training. Many of the things I had Spinks doing, such as lifting weights and running short sprints on a track versus running long distance, were considered unorthodox in boxing training. When Angelo Dundee, Muhammad Ali's trainer, saw what I was doing, he said, "This is crazy. Spinks doesn't stand a chance." Archie Moore, one of the greatest light heavyweight champions of all time, told the press that it couldn't be done: "You don't put muscle on in two months. It takes a lifetime." Moore had tried the same thing and been beaten by heavy-weight boxers Rocky Marciano and Floyd Patterson.

But I knew from my experience working with football players that it *could* be done—and I had the faith and trust of the people with whom I was working. Spinks was a lanky 6' 2" so we had to put a significant amount of extra muscle on his frame to enable him to face up to the 6' 3" Holmes, who at 221½ pounds outweighed him by 21½ pounds. During the eight-week training period, Spinks went from 175 pounds and 9.1 percent body fat to 200 pounds and 7.2 percent body fat. He was ready, both physically and psychologically. Unlike other boxers who come to a fight edgy and hungry because they have been dieting for two months to lose fat weight, he was metabolically energized because I had put him on a high-performance nutrition and supplementation plan.

The night of the Spinks/Holmes fight, Holmes was going for Rocky Marciano's record. If he beat Spinks, he would tie Marciano's record of forty-nine straight wins, the longest winning streak in the history of boxing. Instead, we were the ones who made history. Spinks won a unanimous decision and was declared the new undisputed world heavyweight champion, since defeating Holmes made him the holder of all of Holmes's title division belts. Six months later when Holmes challenged him to a rematch, Spinks won that fight too, reaffirming his tremendous, historically unprecedented achievement.

This victory made me one of the most highly sought after performance enhancement experts in the country. I went on to work with athletes like NBA basketball player Manute Bol of the Washington Bullets (now the Washington Wizards), Ozzie Smith of the St. Louis Cardinals, and Roy Jones Jr., the light heavyweight champion boxer who moved up and beat WBA heavyweight champion John Ruiz on March 1, 2003.

Most recently, I made history again doing the "impossible." Bernard Hopkins, who at age forty-one holds the record for the greatest number of successful middleweight title defenses, wanted to end his career by challenging Antonio Tarver, a younger man, for the light heavyweight championship. To prepare him for this fight, I designed a six-week training program very similar to the one presented in this book. During that time, Hopkins went from 165 pounds to the qualifying weight of 175 pounds. His body fat dropped from 12 percent to 8.75 percent, resulting in a 3.25 percent gain in lean muscle.

On June 10, 2006, Hopkins beat Tarver in a unanimous decision.

Creating the Lean and Hard Study

In 1997, I was approached by Marty Herman, an executive at AmeriFit, a company that manufactures premiere health and wellness supplements. Herman was forming a small advisory board of sports and nutrition experts to create a cutting-edge performance nutrition/supplement program. Herman funded a $30,000 research grant, and we conducted a study at the Louisiana State University Health Care Network, which was then a division of the LSU Medical Center, where I was a full-time clinical health instructor.

This was the only high-performance muscle-development program that I knew of to be tested by a major medical center. It was also the first study of its kind to examine the results of a high-intensity workout coupled with performance nutrition and safe performance supplementation. Other studies had looked at only one of these factors. Our goal was to study the dynamics of these three elements working in tandem.

I made an announcement on my daily radio show that we were looking for twenty volunteers to sign up for this study. We selected a wide cross section of people, ranging from those who never exercised to the superfit who wanted to use our program to increase their already significant lean muscle mass. The participants included an out-of-shape businessman, a high school athlete, a navy SEAL, a homemaker, and a female marathoner. My friend Dr. Jim Flarity, the clinical exercise physiologist who supervised the original Lean and Hard Study, supervised this study. He got a baseline profile on each subject's body composition (ratio of lean muscle to body fat), as well as his or her aerobic fitness, resting heart rate, and overall stamina before beginning the program.

Our aim was to see what could be accomplished in six weeks of high-intensity interval training—lifting weights four days a week, with a day off on Wednesday—for a total of twenty-four workouts. Saturday and Sunday were "recovery days," on which participants could do an optional cardiovascular workout. We also asked our study participants to follow a daily eating plan and a performance nutrition supplementation plan. First, we gave them a complete medical evaluation supervised through the Department of Comprehensive Medicine at Louisiana State University Medical Center. Then we gave them an orientation, the manual describing the high-intensity exercise program and nutrition plan, and a six-week supply of supplements.

What the Study Accomplished

At the end of the Lean and Hard Study, Dr. Flarity retested each subject. The results were amazing. In just six weeks, participants saw significant and startling changes in their bodies. The average study participant experienced the following results:

- A gain of 10 pounds of lean muscle
- A loss of 6 pounds of body fat
- An increase in the efficiency of his or her cardiovascular system (endurance) of 31 percent
- An increase in the efficiency of his or her anaerobic system (stamina) of 13 percent
- A ten-point reduction in his or her resting heart rate
- A dramatic increase in his or her strength and power

This was one of the first studies to demonstrate that even without any cardiovascular training, high-intensity interval training increases endurance. The Lean and Hard Program, which arose from this study, has replicated these results many times since then. In fact, a recent study published in *Medicine and Science in Sports and Exercise* that compared the effects of moderate- and high-intensity training backed up many of the results of my study, for example, the effectiveness of high-intensity training (HIT) over moderate-intensity training (MIT). The study stated: "Despite being matched for total work and producing similar increases in aerobic fitness, 5 weeks of HIT resulted in a significantly greater improvement in RSA (repeated sprint activity) than MIT." The study also showed that the increase in aerobic fitness (or VO2 levels) and rising fatigue levels carried over into *all* areas of sports. No matter who you are or what kind of shape you are in, you can benefit from the program. In as few as twenty-four workouts spread over six weeks, you can begin to get the lean and muscular body you've always wanted.

What This Book Offers

The latest studies in the science of sports medicine show that high-intensity interval training is the quickest way to a muscular physique. Yet there is a great deal of confusion about how to get the most from this type of workout. Many people are also afraid of rigorous exercise programs because they fear that they are not physically fit or knowledgeable enough to handle this kind of a workout. The Lean and Hard Program outlined in this book is so clear, concise, and accessible that anyone can follow it with success. *Lean and Hard* will do the following:

- Give readers a detailed understanding of their bodies' energy and hormonal systems and how to make them more efficient
- Answer questions about effective nutrition for high performance such as "How much protein do I really need?" and "How many calories do I need with a high-performance workout to make sure I am building muscle, not losing it?"
- Explain performance supplementation, providing readers with a simple and safe supplementation program that makes a difference in their workout
- Educate readers about the importance of the recovery phase between high-performance workouts and how to eat and supplement on days between workouts
- Discuss proper hydration before, during, and after high-intensity exercise

Lean and Hard is the ultimate strength-building workout book for those seeking to build the powerful muscular physique they have always dreamed of having. It offers a comprehensive, safe, and intelligent program that can be followed by anyone, whether he or she is a weekend warrior, an athlete, or just an ordinary person who wants to become more buff, lean, and chiseled. This program has worked for a wide variety of people from many walks of life and at different levels of fitness. In this book, I will give you the facts and case histories to prove why this program will work for anyone willing to make a commitment to just twenty-four high-intensity seventy-five-minute workouts—just four workouts a week for six weeks. As with any exercise program, you must consult your doctor before beginning.

My father, who was a combat-decorated captain and company commander in World War II, used to tell me, "Son, you need to train like you fight and fight like you train." Over the years I have modified his words for the thousands of athletes I have worked with, telling them to "Train like you compete in sports and compete like you train." The secret to having the body you want is to train with passion and approach your life with passion. As you age, the lean muscle you gain will pay you dividends in energy, health, and longevity.

PART ONE

Learn the ABCs of High-Intensity Training

1

What Lean Muscle Will Do for You

What Exactly *Is* Lean Muscle?

When we talk about gaining lean muscle, we are really talking about building up and maintaining all the components in the body that are supported by amino acids. Amino acids are the building blocks of your body. They support the critical cell structure not just in your muscles, but also in your internal organs, red blood cells, connective tissue, enzymes that direct metabolism, and antibodies that maintain immune function.

Fat is metabolically inactive—it only serves as a reservoir for excess calories. The body's stores of fat grow or shrink depending upon how active we are and what we eat. Since every protein molecule has a role in maintaining homeostasis, or balance, and health, the body does not have "excess" protein storage. Loss of any body protein is harmful to the body. That is why the high-intensity workout program presented in this book is accompanied by high-performance nutrition and supplementation, so that you will gain lean muscle, not waste it.

Six Benefits of the Lean and Hard Program

Over the years, I have seen the importance of maintaining a healthy level of lean muscle. Being lean and firm not only makes you look better, it improves your performance, your energy levels, and your overall health. Following the Lean and Hard Program can help you achieve the following:

1. Increase your metabolism and energy levels. Fat is something you carry around—it makes you feel tired and metabolically sluggish. Muscle weight carries you around—it is metabolically active. The leaner you are, the more energy you have to perform at your job, play with your children, enjoy life with your spouse, and pursue the sports and creative activities you enjoy.

2. Stop lean muscle loss. Even if your scale weight doesn't change from the time you are twenty years old to the time you are seventy, your body composition is changing. The natural loss of lean muscle (sarcopenia) begins around the age of twenty-five and increases with age. After the age of thirty, most people lose an average of half a pound of muscle and gain about 2½ pounds of fat per year because of the lowered rate of metabolism that muscle loss creates.

The only thing that can stop lean muscle loss is doing weight-bearing exercises—lifting dumbbells, pushing against machines in a gym, or high-intensity interval training—such as those offered in this book.

3. Prolong performance and an active life. Many of the characteristics people associate with aging—being overweight, slowing down, having joint pain, limited mobility, and being less able to do a demanding job—are directly tied to how much lean muscle one has as opposed to body fat. Maintaining and increasing lean muscle mass as you age keeps you active and fully functional.

4. Build your immune system and speed healing. The immune system needs a basic amount of protein to function efficiently. If you have too little lean muscle tissue, your vulnerability to disease and your ability to heal from injury, illness, or surgery can be compromised. Studies have shown that people who have a healthy amount of lean tissue need about 0.8 gram of protein per kilogram (2.2 pounds) of body weight to maintain lean muscle weight. However, people who are undergoing either physical or emotional stress require between 1.5 and 2.0 grams of protein per kilogram to meet the greater metabolic needs placed upon their bodies, which are struggling to repair the damage and normalize all the metabolic processes.

Since most people do not know this, they lose ground during illness—and some never recover from this lean muscle loss. I have a friend who lost 18 pounds undergoing chemotherapy for breast cancer. When she was placed on corticosteroids for six weeks to minimize the negative side effects she was having from a chemotherapy agent, she immediately became ravenously hungry and began gaining back the weight, but it was mostly fat. Her body felt soft and ungainly to her. Now she is working out, eating nutritiously, and taking supplements to transform her body to its former lean and trim shape.

5. Look and feel more youthful. I always tell my clients, "You are as young as you are metabolically active. And you are metabolically active in direct proportion to the amount of lean muscle tissue you have." There is a difference between chronological age and physical age, and gaining lean muscle is one way to turn back the clock. I am fifty-five and my body fat percentage is somewhere between 10 and 12 percent, meaning that most of my weight is lean, metabolically active tissue. The last time I had a physical, my doctor told me that my physical age was nineteen. When I work with athletes, I don't just sit on the sidelines and tell them what to do—I do it with them. And most of the time, even at my age, I can outrun them.

6. Become trimmer. Muscle takes up a third of the space of fat. As you build a higher percentage of lean muscle, your body will become more firm and compact. You may even drop a clothing size while maintaining almost the same scale weight. Sometimes the changes in physique can be dramatic. I have one client who dropped from a size 12 dress to a size 6 after three months of following a performance food program and working out to increase lean muscle. Of course, she lost some weight as well, but her body was dramatically tighter and leaner. She couldn't believe how different she looked.

Lean, Not Skinny

Most people don't realize that there is a dramatic difference between being skinny and being lean. Just because a person's arms, legs, and waistline have a small circumference doesn't mean that he or she is healthy and lean. In fact, many skinny people have a high amount of body fat compared to muscle. This is especially true of sedentary people or those who engage in numerous aerobic activities without any kind of strength training. For example, someone might jog 4 miles a day or swim laps for an hour, yet have a body that looks very skinny and wasted. Cardiovascular activity stimulates little, if any, increase in lean muscle.

Everyone has a certain amount of lean muscle and body fat, but there are healthy and unhealthy percentages. For example, the average body fat percentage for a man is 15 to 17 percent, and lean is considered to be in the range of 11 to 14 percent. For women, 18 to 22 percent is considered average, and 14 to 17 percent is considered lean.

Unless you are a football player loaded with size and muscle, the more body fat you have, the lower your metabolism. You can only increase your metabolic efficiency by increasing your lean muscle mass. The more muscle you have on your frame, the easier it will be to maintain a lean and firm body.

How lean you are has little to do with scale weight. Let's take an example of two men who are both 5' 10" and weigh 220 pounds. The first man is a bodybuilder and has only 7 percent body fat. All the rest of his scale weight, 204.6 pounds, is muscle—metabolically active tissue. His body is lean, firm, and strong. The second man has 35 percent body fat, which is very high for a man. He only has only 143 pounds of metabolically active tissue. His appearance is soft and flabby, he feels sluggish, and he carries a good deal of fat weight in his abdominal area.

The Biggest Misconception about Working Out

Most people believe that if you want to build lean muscle, you must exercise very hard daily. While high-intensity training does demand more effort, it has to be the right kind of effort. The amount of recovery time you allow and your nutritional support are just as important as your workout. Dr. Jim Flarity sums this up well when he says, "It's not just putting in a lot of effort, it's working intelligently. It's difficult to get people to understand that a day of rest can be as important, or more so, than a day of hard training. A day of rest and recovery helps to clear out the lactic acid that exercise creates. Exercise breaks down lean muscle. If you don't allow proper recovery time, when the muscle is challenged again the next day you can overwork it and go backward. Not only will you not improve, you can actually make your body weaker."

The best technique for building lean muscle involves not only the exercise program itself but the time spent recovering from exercise, performance nutrition, and safe, effective performance supplementation.

High-intensity exercise, when done properly, is not about expending energy—it's about learning how to efficiently *manage* your energy. For example, imagine two long-distance runners who are identical in every way. If one expends his greatest effort right out of the starting gate, and the other paces himself, there's no question who will go the distance. The man or woman who learns how to manage his or her energy system—effort, rest and recovery, and nutrition—will receive the greatest gains in lean muscle and strength over time.

And because you will be working out according to your rate of perceived exertion (RPE)—your *subjective* feeling of what level of effort feels light, medium, or hard to you—this program will never overwork your body.

The Ozzie Smith Story

In 1985, I began working with a thirty-year-old baseball player named Ozzie Smith. Earning over two million dollars a year, Ozzie was one of the highest-paid baseball players at that time and had already won a string of Gold Glove awards.

Ozzie felt that he only had a few more years to go in the game, and he wanted to be remembered not just as a great defensive shortstop but as a great all-around player. With a batting average of only 249, he wasn't even considered a hitting threat. He decided

that his only choice was to get bigger and stronger. This was a challenge because, at 154 pounds and 5' 9", he didn't have a lot of size.

While Ozzie was working hard at lifting weights, he did not support his effort with the proper performance nutrition. This really worked against him during the season because he gradually lost weight during the grueling 162-game schedule. By the second half of the season, he had lost 10 pounds and his energy levels and endurance had begun to drop.

When Ozzie told me that he wanted to get a lot bigger, I said, "I know you are a great defensive player. What if I waved a magic wand and gave you a lot more pounds, but you lost your agility and couldn't be a great defensive shortstop anymore? Would you really want that, even if you became a good hitter?"

Ozzie said, "Of course not. Those are the conditions under which I signed my contract. That's what they expect of me."

I told him that our goal would be to build up his body in such a way that he could still do what he already did well. We would use the Lean and Hard Program to hone and maintain his defensive skills, while helping him to develop more strength and power to improve his batting average.

We not only packed on the lean muscle and got his weight up to 172 pounds but also gave him the tools to keep it there for the entire season. Ozzie's transformation was so dramatic that when he showed up at the St. Louis Cardinals' training camp, his teammates couldn't believe their eyes.

Ozzie maintained his weight of 172 all through the season. Not only did he win the Gold Glove, he also won the Silver Bat for his batting average of 303, the best average of a shortstop in baseball that year. He continued to maintain his strength and stamina throughout each ensuing season and raised his overall career batting average to 289.

Instead of the three years he thought he had left, his career continued for another eleven years, until he retired at the age of forty-one. Shortly thereafter, he was inducted into the Baseball Hall of Fame.

You don't have to be a baseball superstar to become lean and hard and gain all the health and lifestyle benefits of building up muscle. If you follow the program presented in this book, you will see dramatic results in body composition and stamina. It works for the top athletes, and it can work for you.

2

Manage Your Hormones to Build Muscle

When we are young, our hormone levels are naturally higher because our bodies are usually lean and our percentage of body fat is low. As we get older, we become less active, shifting our body composition from mostly leaner to fatter. We enter menopause or andropause (male menopause) and our hormone levels drop. If nothing is done to stop this process, every year the average person will gain 2½ pounds of fat and lose 1 pound of lean muscle. This leads to loss of energy, poor body composition, and many health complications.

An important part of getting and staying lean and strong is learning how to enhance your body's ability to manufacture specific types of hormones, which we call "anabolic," because they play an important part in muscle maintenance and growth. A recent article published in the *Journal of Strength and Conditioning* states, "It seems reasonable to suggest that acute exercise-induced responses during HRE [heavy resistance exercise] play an important role in the long-term anabolic adaptation processes related to muscle hypertrophy and maximal strength development, especially during heavy resistance strength training."

There are two basic hormones that influence your capacity to make lean muscle: human growth hormone and insulin. While these hormones decrease with age, inactivity, and fat gain, research has shown that high-intensity training coupled with performance nutrition and supplementation can significantly increase their levels in your body.

Achieve Positive Nitrogen Balance

High-intensity training does not build muscle mass, it breaks down muscle tissue, giving it the *potential* to build itself back up bigger and stronger. This potential is realized if two conditions are met: proper recovery time and proper high-performance nutrition and supplementation.

Carbohydrates stoke your body's furnace, giving you energy to perform during your workout. Maltodextrin is a protein-sparing agent included in this plan. It keeps your body from using its own muscle tissue as energy during your workout.

The protein drinks and supplements you ingest before and after your workout help to repair and increase muscle mass. These high-performance fuels create positive nitrogen balance in your cells. Protein breaks down into amino acids and amino acids break down into nitrogen. When your body has a nitrogen deficit, you will lose muscle mass; when you have a positive nitrogen balance, you will gain muscle mass.

Without the work of anabolic hormones, the body cannot achieve positive nitrogen balance.

The Relationship between Human Growth Hormone and Lean Muscle

Throughout childhood, human growth hormone (HGH) helps to regulate bone and organ growth. In adulthood, it is responsible for many other metabolic processes, including the breakdown and synthesis of protein, which helps create positive nitrogen balance. This means that there is a direct correlation between a person's level of HGH and his or her percentage of lean muscle.

As a person ages, it is natural for levels of HGH to decline gradually, but this drop is significantly increased if one gains body fat and gets little or no exercise. When our doctors test the clients who come into my program, they find that those who have a high percentage of fat and a low percentage of lean muscle have significantly lower than normal levels of HGH. Many people who suffer from a deficiency of HGH can also become depressed, which may lead to feelings of hopelessness about being able to exercise or change their lifestyle for the better. When a person's hormonal levels are low or significantly out of kilter, he or she often finds it difficult to feel motivated.

It is normal for HGH to decrease with age, so no one is going to have the same amount in middle or old age as he or she had in youth. But that does not mean that a person should be resigned to low HGH. What can be done to increase levels of this important anabolic hormone?

A few years back there was a lot of buzz about taking injections of HGH. The media got very excited about this treatment and touted it as the fountain of youth. In a 1990 article in the *New England Journal of Medicine*, Dr. Daniel Rudman presented a pioneering study of HGH supplementation. He found that when he gave HGH supplementation to elderly men, their body fat decreased and their lean muscle mass, overall strength, bone density, and skin thickness increased.

However, interest in injectable HGH began to wane as people found out that it was not the simple solution that it promised to be. In fact, every doctor I asked about HGH injections felt that they were not the answer for several reasons. One is the cost of this therapy—$800 to $1,250 per month—a sum that insurance companies are usually not willing to cover because they don't see a medical necessity for it. Another downside is that it takes up to six months for these injections to begin to take effect. Also, there is the unpleasant prospect of taking a shot four times a week. Sticking yourself with a syringe is not easy. The potential for adverse medical side effects is also a consideration. You must work with your physician to determine whether you are a candidate.

Dr. Michael Murray, a well-known naturopath, warns:

> My take on it is that, like most hormones, it's a double-edged sword and needs to be used very carefully. There's been a lot of publicity about its positive benefits. Not enough press has been given to the potential harmful benefits of excess hormone, such as inducing diabetes and actually promoting the growth of cancer and possibly worsening osteoarthritis. Those are some of the risks of excess growth hormone. I'm not too optimistic that HGH injections will be shown to be all that beneficial in the long term. I believe that taking into consideration diet and lifestyle and trying to maintain natural levels of HGH for as long as possible is the best way to go.

What Are Secretagogues?

In recent years, secretogogues, substances that act like HGH, have appeared on the market. Like HGH injections, these products promise to increase your muscle mass, strength, and bone mass. However, at a recent Consensus Development Conference on Injectable Growth Hormone vs. Growth Hormone Secretogogues hosted by the Great Lakes College of Clinical Medicine, several physicians said that the effectiveness of the products had yet to be shown. Their main concern is that because the products have been around for only three to five years, there simply hasn't been enough time or funding to research their full value.

Secretagogues should not be dismissed out of hand, but they should only be used with your physician's approval. I have successfully used one formula to increase my own levels of HGH—5 grams daily of a powder that contains the amino acids glycine, L-glutamine, L-tyrosine, gaba, L-argenine, pyro glutamic acid, and L-lysine, plus 25 milligrams of anterior pituitary substance. Do be very,

very careful about what kind of secretagogue you take and how often. I take my brand only once or twice a year for a month at a time because I want to avoid any possible negative side effects—and I take it only with my physician's approval. Once I am finished with my course of secretagogues, I always have a follow-up doctor's visit to make sure my health has not been compromised in any way.

The Natural Way to Increase Human Growth Hormone

A number of studies have shown that specific types of exercises done at specific levels of intensity significantly increase the amount of HGH in the body. A recent report in *Exercise and Sport Science Reviews* shows that resistance exercise increases the amount of HGH in subjects. An article in *Strength and Conditioning Journal* stresses the effectiveness of high-intensity interval training in stimulating the production of HGH. These exercises comprise the Lean and Hard Training Program and are discussed in detail in chapter 10.

The Role of Insulin in Creating the Anabolic State

One of the most effective ways to promote metabolic efficiency and gain lean muscle mass is to train the body's ability to manage insulin. Effectively managing insulin is based upon body composition, the glycemic index of the carbohydrates you eat (their complexity and the amount of time it takes to digest them), the types of proteins that you eat, *when* you eat these nutrients in relation to your workout and recovery periods, and the type of exercise you engage in.

Insulin is the hormone involved in storing the energy of the foods that we eat. When there is an overabundance of energy-giving foods in a meal, especially carbohydrates but also proteins and fats, the body will secrete insulin in great quantities. Any nutrients the body cannot use at that time will be stored. Insulin acts upon proteins by promoting amino acid uptake by the cells and the conversion of those amino acids into cell proteins. Insulin converts excess carbohydrates into glycogen, which is stored in the liver and the muscles until it is needed between meals when the body's glucose levels drop. All of the excess carbohydrates that cannot be stored as glycogen are converted into fat and stored in the adipose (fatty) tissues.

Having an unhealthy ratio of lean muscle to body fat leads to a lower metabolic rate and a condition known as insulin resistance. People usually develop a significant loss of lean muscle for three reasons. The first is lifestyle related and can occur at any age—high stress, poor eating habits, and inadequate physical activity. The second, sarcopenia, is the natural wasting of muscle tissue that develops with age in a person who is inactive and does no resistance exercise. The third is cachexia, which is a muscle-wasting condition attributed to severe fever or a disease such as AIDS or cancer.

When a person's lean muscle percentage falls below what is considered healthy, he or she can become insulin resistant. This happens when muscle cells, which make up 30 to 50 percent of the body, get out of shape and lose much of their ability to respond effectively to insulin. This leaves a surplus of glucose in the blood, much more than the body actually needs for its immediate energy needs. In turn, this stimulates the pancreas to release even more insulin to do its job of transporting the glucose through the cell membranes.

Since the fat cells of an overweight individual are more "receptive" to insulin than their muscle cells are, that is where much of the remaining glucose eventually gets deposited. This creates a vicious cycle, causing even more fat gain at the expense of lean muscle.

Train Your Insulin

The strategy for training insulin and regaining and building lean muscle mass is to combine high-intensity interval training with a high-performance diet. This is where the appropriate carbohydrates and protein come in. It is very important for anyone doing high-intensity training to ingest the right types of protein throughout the day.

Protein is a stabilizing food that assists in insulin management, as well as serving other vital roles in normal body function. Getting the right kinds of protein before your workout boosts protein synthesis, amino acid levels, muscle growth, and exercise performance. Protein eaten after the workout, when your body needs it most, is needed for muscle repair and to increase insulin.

To keep insulin levels stable, complex (low-glycemic) carbohydrates should also be consumed throughout the day. However, there is one time when your body can benefit from the right kinds of simple (high-glycemic) carbs. Since muscle glycogen is the primary fuel for high-intensity workouts, especially interval and weight training, your muscles are starved for carbohydrates following your exercise session. This is a good time to create a managed insulin response by consuming a performance nutrition drink containing high-glycemic carbs such as dextrose or maltodextrin, along with whey protein. This controlled elevation in insulin provides the means to shuttle nutrients quickly into muscles to begin recovery and the building of lean muscle mass.

We will discuss high-performance nutrition, performance nutrition drinks, and when you should take them in greater detail later in Part Two.

Testosterone and Lean Muscle

When I talk about anabolic hormones, a lot of people ask, "But what about testosterone? Isn't that the ultimate muscle-building hormone?" While testosterone does play a role in building and maintaining lean muscle, you cannot simply go to your health food store and stock up on bottles of testosterone-enhancing pills.

I had my testosterone levels tested in 1999 when I was noticing the effect of what I suspected was andropause: a drop in energy levels. I went to my doctor to get my levels checked and sure enough, they were far below normal. At the time, I took his suggestion to have the standard testosterone injection. I immediately noticed an increase in my overall muscle mass, libido, and ability to focus and an increase in my level of aggression and energy. However, I knew that getting these shots periodically was not a long-term solution because of the risk of developing an enlarged prostate. With the shot, my testosterone level spiked but did not remain there. It wasn't a cure for the problem.

A year later, in 2000, I had myself retested. My total testosterone value had risen to 417, in the midrange of normal levels and a good 176 points above the lowest testosterone level.

Eventually my levels went back down again. I was extremely disappointed because I had hoped that one testosterone shot would be sufficient. I realized that some kind of lifestyle change was called for if I was to maintain a consistently healthy testosterone level without periodic injections.

The solution was to change my workout to include a higher level of high-intensity training. I switched to interval training on the track instead of a steady-state cardiovascular workout. In the gym, I focused more on full-body movement in weight training so that I was using more of my total muscle mass. I also began to take a supplement containing flower pollen extract, which comes closer than any other plant to mimicking human male hormones. I heard about this supplement twenty years ago from Dr. James Carter, then chairman of the Nutrition Section at the Tulane University School of Public Health and Tropical Medicine. Dr. Carter monitored a study looking for nutrients that could build lean muscle mass in the same manner as anabolic steroids without any of the negative side effects. This study used a well-known bodybuilder as a subject. A certain blend of flower pollen did the job well.

I also increased my intake of zinc. I had read about the effects of zinc on increasing testosterone levels, especially a type called zinc mono-methionine aspartate. I was careful not to exceed 50 milligrams of zinc daily, since larger doses of zinc can lead to copper-deficiency anemia.

By 2002, my total testosterone level had risen from to 273 to 390.6, up 117.6 points. Since then, I've been able to raise it even more. In March 2003, my total testosterone level was 572, even higher than the level I had achieved with my testosterone shot. My mood is now much more balanced and positive, and I find myself able to deal with the physical changes of middle age. Also, my PSA (prostate-specific antigen) level, which is a marker used in prostate screening, has maintained itself at 0.4, which is considered perfectly normal in a healthy male.

Unlike menopause, the drop in hormones that brings on andropause takes ten to fifteen years. One of the benefits of the Lean and Hard Training Program is that it normalizes the levels of all male hormones, which contribute to the maintenance and building of lean muscle mass.

What Happens to Lean Muscle at Menopause?

Estrogen is not an anabolic hormone, but it is more than just a hormone essential for sexual reproduction. Estrogen plays a critical role in maintaining lean muscle, producing red blood cells, promoting healthy neurological function, preventing osteoporosis, and safeguarding the immune system.

Just as women have been conditioned to believe that a certain amount of bone loss is inevitable as their bodies age and begin producing less estrogen, most also believe that they will lose a significant amount of muscle mass in their later years, leading to an inevitable decrease in strength, mobility, and flexibility.

To a large degree, these changes are reversible. The high-intensity training and nutrition plan in this book will help you not only halt the loss of lean muscle but build it back up again. According to an article published in the *Journal of the American Academy of Orthopaedic Surgeons*, most age-related changes in muscle can be reversed through good nutrition and an appropriate exercise program of resistance and strength training.

It used to be that women past the age of fifty were expected to be flabby and out of shape. Women are discovering that even a moderate amount of exercise increases lean muscle volume and makes joints more flexible.

It is never too late to begin exercising. In fact, the *Canadian Journal of Applied Physiology* reports that studies on sarcopenia universally show that older muscle tissue has the same, if not an even *greater* capacity to respond to a vigorous bout of resistance exercise than younger muscle does.

Don't think that just because you are only in your thirties it is too early to begin thinking about preserving your lean muscle. While the average age at which menopause begins is fifty-one, some women begin to experience symptoms such as hot flashes and an increasing waistline measurement as early as age thirty-five.

Testosterone in Women

Testosterone is generally thought of as a male hormone, but it plays an important role in maintaining health, libido, and bone and muscle density in women of all ages.

In puberty, a woman's body begins to produce increased amounts of testosterone because it is the precursor to estrogen. Girls wouldn't become women without testosterone. A woman's levels of testosterone are highest in her early twenties but wane as she ages.

By menopause, since 80 percent of all hormone production decreases, women are usually suffering from a deficiency in estrogen, progesterone, and testosterone. The replacement of estrogen alone does not correct a loss of sex drive, muscle mass, and energy.

Your doctor can perform tests to determine your testosterone levels, and prescribe testosterone replacement therapies such as natural aqueous testosterone lozenges that slowly dissolve in the mouth, testosterone gel that can be applied topically, and the new testosterone patch called Intrinsa.

I am not a strong advocate of hormone replacement therapy. For most women who come into my program suffering from the symptoms of perimenopause or menopause, high-performance exercise, nutrition, and supplementation seem just as effective in addressing these symptoms.

Just as research has shown that a high-intensity training (HIT) workout increases all levels of anabolic hormones in men, studies have shown that the same prescription works just as well to increase levels of estrogen, progesterone, and testosterone in women.

Angela: How High-Intensity Training Increased Her Anabolic Hormones

I saw how high-intensity training, nutrition, and performance supplementation worked for one woman named Angela. She came to my program because she read about how we helped men and women develop greater muscle tone and strength, and she hoped we could do the same for her.

Angela, fifty-six, had been in menopause for five years and had really gotten out of shape. As many women do when they find their libido on the wane, she told herself that sex really wasn't that important anymore.

Her husband, a dynamic CEO of a major company, didn't feel the same way and began to look elsewhere for sexual relationships. Angela came to this program to save both her marriage and her health. She was a striking woman, but years of losing lean muscle, gaining fat, not exercising, and eating poorly had taken all of the sparkle out of her. She was tired all the time, felt depressed, and slept poorly.

The most remarkable part of Angela's story was how an HIT program made her feel. When she came into the program, she had a low libido and little self-esteem. After only one month, she told me, "I have so much energy and feel so much better, it's like I'm a whole new woman." As her body transformed into a leaner and harder version, her confidence levels soared, and she began to feel more open to life than she ever had before. Not only did her sexual relations with her husband improve, but she felt as if she could be more open and honest with him.

Most important, she told me that for the first time in her life she felt like his equal. "This program not only transformed my inner self, but it transformed me as a person. It made me realize that I could do something to effect change." Angela moved from being a homemaker who always put other people's needs before her own to a person who could create change for herself—and she felt wonderful.

Start Early

As a performance enhancement consultant to many top professional and industrial athletes, I prepare my clients for any contingency. When I explain to them the importance of taking preventative measures, I often use the world of boxing as an example. When I prepare a boxer to defend his title or take another, it is essential that I teach him to anticipate how his opponent will attack him so that he can avoid those punches as often as possible.

You, too, want to avoid those punches. There are certain physical and hormonal changes that will occur as you get older. You know your opponent; start fighting back.

What the Experts Say about Creating the Anabolic State

When I wanted to learn about building and maintaining lean muscle, I didn't just turn to the science of sports medicine. I studied the literature written about AIDS, cancer, and burn patients, for whom lean muscle percentage can mean the difference between life and death. There is no other group of people more likely to lose lean muscle and more in need of getting it built back up again quickly.

As we saw in chapter 1, "What Lean Muscle Will Do for You," the body has no excess protein stores. Energy management and preservation of lean muscle take on new meaning when the body is severely depleted. If a person loses 40 percent of his or her protein stores, death will almost always result.

In order for people with severe injuries or wounds following surgery to heal in a timely fashion, medical experts say they need three things:

1. To eat enough of the right kind of food calories—including complex carbohydrates, appropriate fats, and sufficient protein—to meet the energy demands that the stress of healing places upon their body
2. Sufficient micronutrients in the form of supplements to optimize their metabolism
3. To receive anabolic hormones to help restore lean mass and improve healing

As you can see, the metabolic prescription given to people whose protein stores and energy need replenishing during the stress of recovery from serious injury or illness is very similar to the program I have designed to build up your lean muscle after your sessions of high-intensity exercise.

This kind of research, about building muscle tissue, hormones, and metabolism through nutrition, exercise, and targeted supplementation, has been invaluable to trainers and performance fitness consultants. The same principles apply when designing a program to add lean muscle mass, strength, and power to a professional athlete.

Brett Butler: Returning to the Sport He Loved

In my thirty-year career, I have helped thousands of athletes to build stamina and lean muscle. No story is more dramatic than that of the baseball legend Brett Butler. With the help of his doctors, I designed a high-intensity exercise and performance nutrition and supplementation program to help Brett regain the muscle he lost during cancer treatments and return to baseball, something that his doctors said couldn't be done.

In May 1996, Brett had fifty lymph nodes removed from his neck and throat. One of them was cancerous. Since I had worked with him for the previous eight years and was a close friend, I was one of the first people he called when he learned he had cancer. Brett's ultimate goal was to live, but to him that meant being able to play baseball again. I told him I'd do everything in my power to help him.

After his doctors and I had assessed Brett's health, we went to work building back the lean muscle he lost following his surgery and extensive radiation treatments. At 5' 9", he normally weighed 165 pounds. During his illness, he had lost 20 pounds of muscle. Our goal was to return him to his anabolic state. I had plenty of experience helping tall, thin NBA players gain weight after they burned off the pounds during the basketball season. With Brett, however, there was an additional problem. His radiation treatments made his throat swell and develop sores. How were we going to build him back up if he couldn't swallow solid food?

We found our answer one afternoon while sitting in the doctors' dining room at the hospital. A radiologist at our table said, "When we have to desensitize the throat to put something down it, such as a tube, we numb it with a special medication." I asked him if he would call the pharmacist and order some for Brett. He agreed and Brett began gargling with the medication before meals. It worked perfectly, and he was able to swallow food again without pain.

We created a special drink containing a high-calorie combination of complex carbohydrates, protein powder, and creatine monohydrate to increase his lean muscle mass. Brett drank this three times a day between meals and slowly began to gain back the weight and muscle mass he had lost.

Once Brett became strong enough to begin exercising again, I created a special high-intensity resistance and interval training program for him. Since his surgery had left him with impaired nerve function, I hooked up his shoulder to a monitor to make sure that we were never overtiring his nerves or his muscles. I also got him back into baseball-related activities. The New Orleans Zephyrs' triple-A baseball team gave him permission to do batting practice with them.

The results were remarkable. Brett gained back 17 pounds of lean muscle in twenty-three days, and over a six-week period, his immune function and blood levels improved dramatically. He was able to return to his team, open the series in Montreal, then go home to a standing ovation in Dodger Stadium. He scored the winning run that night. Sports commentators referred to that season as "the amazing comeback." Brett eventually wrote about his recovery in a book called *Field of Hope*, in which he devoted an entire chapter to the work we had done together. As of this writing, he is still cancer free.

PART TWO

The Lean and Hard Nutritional Program

3

Performance Nutrition

Eat to Build Muscle and Increase Metabolism

A high-intensity workout requires a high-performance nutritional program. You would not put the fuel you use in your Ford Taurus into the car you want to drive in the Indy 500. Likewise, if you want to become lean and hard, you cannot eat the way you always have or your body will lack sufficient energy to build your physique.

Many people make the mistake of decreasing their caloric intake at the same time they begin an HIT program. They think that too much food made them fat in the first place, so eating less will melt the fat and the intense exercise will build more lean muscle.

The opposite is true. If you attempt to go on a calorically restrictive diet while exercising intensely, you will not build muscle but will instead break down muscle as your body searches for fuel reserves. If you want your body to remain in the anabolic state during and after your workout, you must ingest not only *more* calories each day than you normally do but the *right kind* of calories. This includes a greatly increased amount of lean protein, the right kind of carbohydrates at the right time, and the proper amount of unsaturated and monounsaturated fats.

Five Benefits of Performance Nutrition

High-performance nutrition can enhance your workout in five ways:

1. It can inhibit the breakdown of lean muscle (catabolism) during your training session.
2. It can improve protein synthesis (anabolism). When the body is properly fueled, it is in positive nitrogen balance, which promotes the building of lean muscle mass.
3. It can increase muscle energy production and delay fatigue. A substance called phosphocreatine is stored in the muscle cells until it is needed to produce the molecule known as adenosine triphosphate, or ATP, which powers the body and causes muscular contraction. The ATP molecule has three phosphates attached to it. When one of these phosphates breaks lose, energy is released. In order for your body to create more ATP, it must have an abundance of phosphates ready to reattach to the depleted molecules.
4. It can change your body composition by increasing lean muscle weight and reducing body fat in conjunction with the high-intensity training program. The Lean and Hard Study showed that over six weeks, participants gained an average of 10 pounds of muscle mass and lost an average of 6 pounds of fat.
5. It can accelerate recovery time. One of the keys to rapid muscle gain is optimizing nutrition during recovery time. The performance nutrition plan is designed to ensure that your body is fully recovered before your next high-intensity workout.

Eating for High Performance

Athletes often ask me, "How much protein, carbohydrate, and fat should I ingest to support my workout?" The answer varies according to the type of activity, the level of training, the length of each session, and the sport the athlete plays.

Here is a list of some sports and the average caloric requirements of an individual in training for them. Notice that the bodybuilding program requires the greatest amount of protein.

Sport	Calories	Protein	Fat	Carbohydrates
Basketball	5,500	1,650	1,100	2,750
Boxing	5,800	1,740	1,160	2,900
Sprinting	5,200	1,560	1,040	2,600
Bodybuilding	6,800	2,040	1,360	3,400

Of course, if you actually tried to get all of these calories from food alone, you would be eating all day long. That is why you will be ingesting high-calorie performance nutrition drinks before, during, and after your workout, and before you go to bed at night. These drinks will enable you to follow the three R's of performance nutrition: replace, recover, and repair.

This program uses two basic types of drinks:

1. A good whey protein drink containing sufficient essential (not made by the body) and nonessential (made by the body) amino acids to help repair the body and build muscle
2. Drinks containing substances such as creatine, glutamine, and maltodextrine, which can help to increase lean muscle mass and accelerate recovery between workouts. Maltodextrin is such a concentrated source of carbohydrate that one cup contains the same amount of energy found in six plates of whole-wheat pasta.

If you want to repair tissue and build muscle mass, the timing of your meals and performance nutrition drinks is as important as *what* and *how much* you eat. This book is one of the few that gives you a complete, day-by-day, workout-by-workout nutritional and supplemental script to help you fuel for your workout, recover from it, and maximize your lean muscle gains.

Getting enough protein is extremely important because it is the structural basis of all body tissues. The amino acids found in protein are the building blocks of life, involved in the growth and repair of muscle, and the enzymes found in proteins regulate all metabolic processes. Protein and amino acids support your ability to train at a level that increases strength, power, stamina, and endurance.

The Importance of High-Quality Proteins

To support your high-intensity training, I suggest a daily lean protein intake of 1.2 to 1.6 grams per kilogram (2.2 pounds) of body weight if you are female, and 1.4 to 1.8 grams per kilogram if you are male. This may sound a bit complicated, but I will do all the food calculations for you in chapter 5, "Lean and Hard Meal Plans for High Performance." Good sources of protein are chicken breasts, all types of fish, beef with a low fat content (in moderation), soy products, and whey products.

Protein is stored on a limited basis, so people undergoing high-intensity training require three balanced meals and three snacks that include the proper level of protein per day to enable them to maximize their workout, achieve adequate recovery, and increase muscle mass.

When choosing protein sources, always choose lean meats, fish, and low-fat dairy. First-choice protein sources include 95 percent lean ground beef or turkey, skinless chicken breasts, white-meat tuna in water, egg whites, fish and seafood (baked or grilled, never fried), skim milk, fat-free cheese and cottage cheese, and yogurt made from skim milk.

I always suggest that clients eat cold-water fish such as salmon and halibut at least twice a week, or even once daily if they really love fish. According to the *American Journal of Clinical Nutrition*, eating fish daily stabilizes levels of the anabolic hormone insulin, increases glucose production, lowers triglyceride (bad fat) production, and increases the level of HDL (good) cholesterol, reducing the risk of cardiovascular disease.

Many people are concerned today about the dangers of mercury in fish. This is a serious issue, especially if you have children in your family. Generally, you should avoid eating fish such as swordfish, tilefish, and king mackerel more than once a week since these larger oceangoing fish have accumulated larger concentrations of mercury in their bodies. When it comes to tuna, albacore has the highest level of mercury. If you want to give your family a tuna fish sandwich, choose light tuna, which has very low mercury concentrations. Cold-water fish such as freshwater mackerel, cod, and sardines are also safe sources of protein.

The Benefits of Soy

Soy products have always been a part of my nutritional programs because of their many benefits. Research has shown that an overabundance of the amino acid lysine increases the level of bad cholesterol in the body, while the amino acid arginine decreases it. Compared to animal protein, soy has a more favorable ratio of arginine to lysine. This lower ratio helps the body to balance its production of insulin and increase its production of glucagon. Eating soy frequently helps you to shift your metabolism from fat storage to production of lean muscle mass.

Besides soy-based powders, there are many delicious soy food products available, including soy burgers and hot dogs, tofu, soy cheese, and soy milk. Since one of the challenges faced by vegetarians is getting sufficient protein in their daily diet, soy products can be a nutritional mainstay.

Carbohydrates: Energy for Your High-Intensity Workout

You won't get the full benefit of the protein you ingest without the protein-sparing agent: carbohydrates. They are an energy engine, powering your workout and recovery and allowing your body to use all of its available protein sources to repair and build muscle. Research has shown that you can best support a high-intensity workout using a 4:1 ratio of carbohydrate to protein.

In the arena of high-intensity training, a popular slogan is "Protein is king." But if you really want to spare protein during and after your workout, using your available stores to pack on the muscle, then carbohydrates are the crown prince.

In recent years, carbohydrates have gotten a bad name. This is unfortunate, because complex (slow-digesting) carbohydrates are the most efficient fuel source for the body during high-intensity training. Adequate carbohydrate intake and proper timing will help you to get the most out of your high-intensity workout.

In his book *The Handbook of Sports Nutrition*, John Williams, who designed the high-performance supplementation protocol for this book, describes how carbohydrate works in the body:

> Carbohydrate is processed by the digestive system and liver, converted into glucose and released into the bloodstream, which causes a rise in blood sugar. This sudden rise in blood sugar triggers the pancreas to release the hormone insulin. To lower the blood sugar level, insulin acts to transport the glucose into various tissues, primarily muscle cells and the liver. If there is an excess of carbohydrate it is conveniently stored as fat. . .
>
> Blood glucose is the primary source of fuel for the central nervous system including the brain. When the blood glucose level drops too low (hypoglycemia) a person will feel weak and unstable. To prevent the onset of hypoglycemia, the body converts liver glycogen into glucose. Unfortunately, the liver glycogen stores are relatively small and cannot sustain an endurance activity.

When a person is involved in high-intensity activities requiring short bursts of intense energy, such as the Lean and Hard Training Program, his or her muscle glycogen stores will be rapidly depleted, resulting in fatigue. Therefore, the high-performance nutrition and supplementation programs described in this book are designed to keep adequate levels of carbs in your body when you need their energy the most.

Eating the right amount of complex carbohydrates throughout the day will help to keep your levels of blood sugar from fluctuating and stabilize levels of the anabolic hormone insulin. This will maintain balanced energy and promote a leaner, more muscular physique.

To support your high-intensity workout and recovery process, ingest 4 to 6 grams of carbohydrate per kilogram (2.2 pounds) of body weight daily. Since I am not asking you to do an endurance workout, this number is the same for both males and females.

Carbohydrates That Support High-Intensity Training

An important criterion to keep in mind when choosing appropriate carbohydrates is their rating on the glycemic index. Foods with a high-glycemic rating (simple sugars) stimulate a higher than normal production of insulin in the body and tend to stimulate fat storage, except when taken first thing in the morning and during or right after a workout. Foods that have a low-glycemic rating (complex carbohydrates) digest slowly and do not significantly elevate insulin but rather keep insulin levels steady throughout the day.

Examples of simple carbohydrates are potatoes, white bread, bananas, white rice, pancakes, desserts, sugary soft drinks, pizza, and candy. Complex carbohydrates include yams, sweet potatoes, brown rice, whole-grain cereals, bran or flaxseed muffins, apples, and oatmeal.

There are three times during the day when consuming high-glycemic (simple, fast-digesting) carbohydrates works to your advantage. The first is right after you awaken in the morning after ten or more hours of not eating. Ingesting some simple carbohydrates first thing in the morning will quickly refuel your muscles with little risk of these carbs being stored as fat. The wisest strategy is to also include some complex carbohydrates with this meal to help stabilize insulin and blood sugar levels after your muscle glycogen has been restored. An example of this kind of breakfast would be oatmeal (complex carb) with some fruit and honey (simple carbs) along with some protein, such as a hard-boiled egg.

The second time when it is advantageous to consume simple carbohydrates is during your workout. Maltodextrin in moderation dissolved in a sports drink such as Gatorade is a good choice. This keeps your energy levels high so that whatever protein you have in your body can be used entirely to build and repair muscle tissue. I explain how to take maltodextrine in chapter 7, "The Lean and Hard Daily Performance Nutrition Supplementation Schedule."

You should also ingest simple carbohydrates right after your high-intensity workout, when your muscle glycogen is depleted and you need a quick burst of simple sugar to refill the tank. Drinks containing simple carbohydrates, such as Powerade or Gatorade, are your best choices at such times.

Chapter 4, "The Lean and Hard Food Exchange List," includes examples of high- and low-glycemic carbs. For a more extensive list of these carbs, please see my book *Lose Your Love Handles*.

Fats: Another Important Energy Source

Second to carbohydrates, fats are another great energy source. Fats are stored in the body in the form of triglycerides. During moderate- to high-intensity exercise, triglycerides are broken down into glycerol and free fatty acids, which are transported to the mitochondria (powerhouse) of the cell. During low-intensity exercise and rest, fats contribute 50 to 60 percent of the body's energy demands. To support your workout and recovery process, I suggest ingesting 0.8 to 1 gram of fat per kilogram (2.2 pounds) of body weight daily.

A good HIT program will actually increase your body's ability to use healthy fats as an energy source and the following will result:

- Your muscles will develop the ability to more efficiently use fats (and carbohydrates) as an energy source.

- Oxidizing fats at a faster rate will enable your body to substitute fat for carbohydrate as an energy source at a specific level of workout intensity.
- Your newfound ability to more efficiently utilize fats will spare your muscle glycogen stores, keeping you in the anabolic state and increasing your energy and endurance.

Good fats, such as the essential fatty acids omega-3 and omega-6, also have a number of health benefits. They protect vital organs and can lower cholesterol, improve joint health, reduce inflammation, and help protect against cancer. Even though it seems counter to logic, ingesting the right kinds of fat actually enables you to use dietary fat to help *burn* body fat.

The Three Kinds of Fat

There are three different groups of fat: saturated fats, trans-fatty acids, and monounsaturated fats such as omega-3 and omega-6.

Saturated fats should only be eaten in limited amounts because they can raise your cholesterol, increasing your chances of heart disease. People who eat diets high in saturated fats also run a greater risk of developing diabetes and some kinds of cancers. These types of fat are found in meats such as beef and pork and dairy products such as cheese and butter.

Trans-fatty acids pose an even greater threat to your health. They are formed when vegetable or fish oils are hydrogenated. French fries, doughnuts, cookies, chips, and other snack foods are all high in trans-fatty acids. In fact, nearly all fried or baked goods have some trans-fat content.

The best kind of fat to include in your diet is monounsaturated fat, found in plant products such as olive oil (omega-9), canola oil, nuts, and avocados. Your body uses this type of fat to strengthen cell membranes, support nerve and hormone function, and produce hormonelike substances called prostaglandins, which have been linked to the prevention of heart disease and cancer.

Essential Fatty Acids Decrease Health Risks

Two kinds of unsaturated fats are necessary for your survival. These are the essential fatty acids omega-6 (linoleic acid) and omega-3 (linolenic acid). Since your body cannot manufacture these fatty acids, they must be obtained from the foods you eat. Omega-6 is fairly common and is found in most vegetable oils. Remember that it is better to buy your oils in amber or green bottles, since exposure to sunlight destroys freshness and can make oils become rancid. It is also better to buy oils in health food stores if you can. Many typical grocery store oils, which are processed for mass distribution, are filled with free radicals—short-lived, highly reactive chemicals often derived from oxygen-containing compounds, which can have detrimental effects on cells, particularly DNA and cell membranes—and trans-fatty acids.

Omega-3 is found in soy; walnut, flax, fish, and canola oils; and dark green, leafy vegetables. It is especially important to make sure that you supplement your food plan with enough omega-3 fats, since the American diet is usually deficient in this nutrient. While the ideal ratio of omega-6 oil to omega-3 is between 3:1 and 4:1, a recent study showed that most people have twenty times the level of omega-6 than omega-3.

Ten Benefits of "Good" Fats

There are many benefits to eating the proper amount of unsaturated fats and essential fatty acids. These good fats can do the following:

1. Provide an excellent source of energy for your high-intensity workout
2. Reduce free radicals
3. Lower total cholesterol levels by preventing platelet aggregation (blood clotting), and vasoconstriction, or blood vessel constriction
4. Lower triglycerides
5. Raise levels of high-density lipoprotein (good) cholesterol
6. Lower high blood pressure
7. Decrease symptoms of heart palpitations, also known as angina
8. Lower the risk of heart attacks and strokes
9. Decrease the pain and swelling of rheumatoid arthritis
10. Lower the risk for many types of cancer, including breast cancer

How to Increase the Essential Fatty Acids in Your Diet

There are several ways to increase the amount of essential fatty acids in your diet. For example, cold-water fish such as salmon, mackerel, and trout are rich sources of the essential fatty acid metabolites DHA (docosahexaenoic acid) and EPA (eicosapentaenoic acid). Aside from simply eating fish at least twice per week, you can supplement your diet with omega-3 by taking fish oil capsules, which are available at most pharmacies or health food stores.

Flax oil is another rich source of omega-3 and all other essential fatty acids, which is why bodybuilders mix it into their protein drinks so often. It is best taken in liquid form rather than in capsules to ensure that it is fresh and of high quality. The next time you are fixing a green salad, try using a tablespoon of flax oil as a dressing, or half a tablespoon of flax oil mixed with sunflower oil or a little vinegar. You may also lightly brush it over meat after the meat has been cooked. Mixing flax oil with low-fat cottage cheese helps your body use the oil, since the sulfur content of cottage cheese enhances its effectiveness.

Ground flaxseed, which you can sprinkle over your breakfast cereal or salad or blend into a protein drink, is another great source of omega-3.

Other Sources of Unsaturated Fats

Other acceptable sources of unsaturated fats include Hellman's Light Mayonnaise, Kraft Light Mayonnaise, Smart Balance Soft Spread (no trans-fatty acids), and unsaturated corn oil. Products such as Promise, Take Control, Fleischmann's Margarine, and I Can't Believe It's Not Butter (spray, not solid) are excellent butter alternatives. If real butter is your only alternative when dining out, use it in moderation.

How I Packed the Pounds onto the Basketball Star Manute Bol

When I met the 7' 7" Washington Bullets star Manute Bol, he was the tallest player in the NBA. He was so tall he'd had the front seat of his Ford Bronco removed and drove it from the backseat. At 195 pounds, he was seriously underweight relative to his physical requirements for the NBA, a problem that negatively affected his performance and his endurance. Manute needed to put on some muscle weight fast or he wasn't going to make it through the season.

Unfortunately, everything he and his camp had tried so far had failed to do the job, including hiring a well-known strength coach. Abe Polan, who owned the Washington Bullets and treated Manute like his own son, made me an offer. He would pay me for every pound I put on Manute.

I asked Abe if I could see where Manute lived because I wanted to get an idea of his eating habits and the way things were set up in his living space. Manute came from the Dinka tribe in Sudan, Africa. In his tribe, only women cooked, so even in this country all of Manute's food was brought to his home, already prepared.

When I saw the setup in his apartment, I couldn't understand why Manute was not gaining weight. His refrigerator was certainly full of food. Then I did something other people hadn't—I began to closely observe his daily life and ask him questions. One of the first things I noticed as we shared some meals together was that he wouldn't eat salads or vegetables. When I asked him why, he said, "This food tastes strange to me."

I soon discovered that Manute did not put his food away immediately, but would open all of the containers, sample the different foods, then leave everything in the kitchen while he ate and did other things. Eventually, he would remember to seal everything up and put it away in the refrigerator. By that time, the food would be spoiled.

Now that I understood what the problem was, I took Manute with me back to New Orleans and put him on a program very similar to the one described in this book. I fed him over 7,500 calories a day, divided between three main meals (which added up to approximately 3,000 calories), four snacks, and performance nutrition supplementation before, during, and after his workout sessions and before bedtime.

To help design the supplementation part of Manute's program, I consulted with my longtime friend and colleague, the sports performance nutrition expert John Williams. We made sure that Manute got plenty of amino acids and maltodextrin before his workout; a carbohydrate drink made with maltodextrin during his workout so that he wouldn't use up his own body stores of carbohydrate; and more maltodextrin in his whey protein shake after his workout. Manute loved apple juice, so I mixed a balanced blend of whey protein and carbohydrate powders to stabilize his insulin level and stimulate his appetite, added it to apple juice, and kept pitchers of the juice in his refrigerator.

Counting all of the meals, snacks, and performance nutrition supplementation Manute received, he was eating ten times a day (not counting the maltodextrin mixed with apple juice he drank during his workouts). He'd have a hearty breakfast, then eat before his workout, after his workout, before lunch, at lunch, before his afternoon workout, after his afternoon workout, before dinner, at dinner, and before bedtime. He was staying in a hotel and I had all his food sent in to him.

Following a high-performance nutrition plan, a performance nutrition supplementation program, and a rigorous program of resistance training similar to the Lean and Hard Training Program, Manute slowly began to pack on the muscle and weight. I had him working out four days a week, playing basketball five days a week, and resting on the weekends.

Over a six-week period, Manute went from 195 pounds to 236 pounds, which resulted in a gain of 38 pounds of lean muscle. Abe; the team general manager, Bob Ferry; and the team doctors and trainers were amazed. When Manute came back to Washington, they brought him to their fitness laboratory to check him out to make sure that he hadn't lost any strength or flexibility. They discovered that not only was he stronger and more flexible, but his added pounds were pure lean muscle as opposed to fat.

I took home a great paycheck, and Abe got what he had hoped for: an athlete who had strength, stamina, and muscle.

4

The Lean and Hard Food Exchange List

The Right Proteins, Carbohydrates, and Fats

As we discussed in the previous chapter, a sound muscle-gain program requires more than just high-intensity exercise. Proper nutrition is also crucial.

Lean and Hard Nutrition Basics

Your high-performance nutrition program will change the way you've probably been eating. Instead of having three meals a day, you should eat five to six smaller meals and snacks throughout the day. Smaller, frequent meals provide the body with the proper fuel it needs to achieve optimal muscle growth and development. In addition, you will see an improvement in your resting energy expenditure (metabolism). Frequent meals, when combined with exercise, are easier on the system and will assist in burning off excess body fat. Don't skip meals, as this leads to the potential use of muscle tissue for energy and causes muscle breakdown, lowering your metabolism and decreasing your lean muscle mass.

We've discussed that carbohydrates are critical for the success of this program. Fueling your body with the right kind of carbohydrates is essential to achieving optimal energy levels during exercise and proper recovery following exercise. Doing this will also help you to use protein effectively to gain lean muscle. The type and amount of carbohydrates you eat will help determine how your body adapts to your training regimen. Also, think about *when* you have your carbohydrates (see below).

As we discussed in chapter 3, "Performance Nutrition," carbohydrates can be classified as either low glycemic or high glycemic.

- **Low-glycemic** carbohydrates are slow digesting and help to control blood sugar and insulin levels throughout the day, promoting satiety (fullness) after meals. Whole grains, fresh fruit and vegetables, and low-fat dairy products are considered low-glycemic carbohydrates. It is a good idea to eat mostly low-glycemic carbs *before your workout to stabilize your blood sugar*.
- **High glycemic** carbohydrates are *essential after the workout when muscles are recovering*. They provide a rapid rise in blood sugar and insulin levels that are critical after exercise to replenish depleted muscle glycogen levels.

Proper hydration is also key. It is important for cellular metabolism, optimal performance, energy balance, and recovery following exercise. In addition, proper fluid intake is required for the absorption of the water-soluble vitamins (B and C). I recommend that each day you consume between ½ and 1 ounce of fluid for every pound of body weight. For example, a person weighing 150 pounds should drink between 75 and 150 ounces of fluid. Proper fluid intake includes water, 100 percent fruit juice, and low-fat milk. While some people may wish to count soft drinks and beverages containing caffeine toward their daily required fluid intake, these are very poor choices, and I do not recommend them. Remember, caffeine is a diuretic.

Also, be mindful that excessive alcohol intake can impair your exercise performance in a variety of ways. Alcohol consumption inhibits protein synthesis, which inhibits muscle growth. On the other hand, moderate alcohol consumption has been proven to decrease your risk of heart disease and may lower blood pressure by reducing stress levels. I recommend that women consume no more than one drink per day and men no more than two drinks.

Calculating Recommended Daily Calories

When following a high-performance muscle-building program, you will need to significantly increase the number of calories you eat daily to give your body the fuel it needs to exercise and increase muscle mass. Generally, the recommended diet for most athletes is approximately 2,500 to 3,000 calories a day, excluding performance nutrition supplementation (see chapter 6, "Lean and Hard Performance Supplementation"). However, since the caloric requirements of a

200-pound man and a 135-pound woman are significantly different, I am going to give you a formula to determine how many calories you should ingest daily.

The best way to determine how many calories your body actually needs is by estimating your total daily caloric (energy) expenditure. This figure will include your resting metabolic rate (RMR)—the number of calories required for basic bodily processes such as tissue repair, brain function, blood circulation, and digestion, and so on—plus the number of calories burned during exercise and normal daily activity.

Step 1: Determine Your Resting Metabolic Rate

If you are a woman, use the following formula to determine your RMR:

$$655 + (\text{weight in kg} \times 9.6) + (\text{height in cm} \times 1.8) - (\text{age} \times 4.7)$$

To convert pounds to kilograms, divide them by 2.2. To convert inches to centimeters, multiply them by 2.5. For example, if you are a forty-year-old woman who weighs 125 pounds and is 5' 6" tall, you would divide 125 by 2.2 to get 56.8 kg. Then you would multiply 66 inches times 2.5 to get a height of 165 cm. You would then get out your calculator and plug those figures into the equation to get your RMR.

$$\text{Weight: } 56.8 \text{ kg} \times 9.6 = 545.28$$
$$\text{Height: } 165 \text{ cm} \times 1.8 = 297$$
$$\text{Age: } 40 \text{ years} \times 4.7 = 188$$
$$\text{Finally: } (655 + 545.28 + 297) - 188 = 1{,}309 \text{ calories (RMR)}$$

If you are a man, use this formula to compute your RMR:

$$66 + (\text{weight in kg} \times 13.7) + (\text{height in cm} \times 5) - (\text{age} \times 6.8)$$

Since these formulas factor in gender, weight, height, and age, they are very precise and should be your preferred method for determining your RMR. However, if the math seems too much for you, a simple way to approximate your RMR is to multiply your body weight by 10. Using this formula, the 125-pound woman mentioned above has a resting metabolic rate of 1,309 calories.

Step 2: Calculate the Number of Calories You Need to Support Your Workout

Once you have calculated your RMR, the next thing you need to do is to calculate how many calories you will need to support your high-intensity workout. The formula I use is the following:

If you are male: $\text{RMR} \times 2.1$ = number of calories you should ingest daily

If you are female: $\text{RMR} \times 1.9$ = number of calories you should ingest daily

Again, let's use our forty-year-old, 125-pound woman. As you saw above, when we calculated her RMR, we got 1,309 calories. That's the amount of food she would need to support her metabolism if all she did was lay in bed all day and do nothing. If we want to see how many calories she would need to perform high-intensity training four days per week, we plug her RMR into the formula:

$$1,309 \text{ calories (RMR)} \times 1.9 = 2,487 \text{ calories}$$

That's how many calories she should eat to manage her energy efficiently during her high-intensity workouts and repair and build muscle. You can see why people who join a gym and then begin to starve themselves to gain muscle and lose fat soon get into trouble. Without proper caloric support for your workout two things will happen. The first is that instead of getting hard, your muscles will become soft and mushy since your body will begin to cannibalize them to get enough protein to sustain your metabolism. The second is that you will be likely to injure yourself because you will be too weak to handle the exercise requirements. Check with a licensed nutritionist to assist with the design of your meal plan, if you choose.

Nutrient Exchange List

Now that you know how many calories you should ingest daily during your HIT, the next step is to plan your meals. The chart below gives you a general idea of how many "exchanges" (precise portions of a food) you will need to meet your caloric requirement. You will find an extensive list of food exchanges below, followed by some suggested meal plans organized according to daily caloric needs.

NUTRIENT EXCHANGES

Calories	1,500	1,800	2,000	2,200	2,500	3,000	3,500	4,000	4,500
Starch (no. of exchanges)	6–8	8–10	10–12	11–13	12–14	14–16	16–18	18–20	19–21
Milk (no. of exchanges)	2	2	2	2	3	3	3	3	5
Fruit (no. of exchanges)	4	4–5	5	5	6	6	7	7	8
Vegetable (no. of exchanges)	3	3	3	3	4	6	7	8	9
Fat (no. of exchanges)	0	0	2	2	3	4	5	5	6
Lean Meat (no. of exchanges)	6–8	8–10	9–11	9–11	10–12	12–14	14–16	16–17	18–20
Percent Carbohydrate	63	57	56	58	58	58	60	62	61
Percent Protein	24	28	29	27	27	25	25	18	20
Percent Fat	13	15	15	15	15	15	15	20	19

Foods are divided into six different groups because they vary in their carbohydrate, protein, and calorie content. Each exchange list includes foods that are alike—they contain about the same amount of carbohydrate, protein, fat, and calories.

The following chart shows the amount of these nutrients in one serving from each exchange list.

NUTRIENTS IN EXCHANGES

Unit	Carbohydrate (grams)	Protein (grams)	Fat (grams)	Calories
Starch/Bread	15	0–3	Trace	80
Meat				
Lean		7	3	55
Medium Fat		7	5	75
High Fat		7	8	100
Vegetable	5	2	—	25
Fruit	15	—	—	60
Milk				
Skim	12	8	Trace	90
Low Fat	12	8	5	120
Whole	12	8	8	150
Fat	—	—	5	45

As you read the exchange list, you will notice that one "exchange" is often a larger amount of food than another choice from the same list. Because foods are so different, each food is measured or weighed so that the amount of carbohydrate, protein, fat, and calories is the same in each choice.

If you have a favorite food that is not included in any of these groups, ask your dietitian about it. Specific high-sodium foods may be worked into your meal plan when consumed in moderation.

General Nutrition Guidelines

1. Try to eat five or six times a day (snacks and main meals). Take at least twenty minutes to eat your main meals.
2. Drink ½ to 1 ounce of *water* per pound of body weight each day. Beverages containing caffeine, alcohol, and sugar do not count toward

this total. Be especially sure to drink enough water to balance your losses through perspiration during your workout or during hot summer months.

3. Select whole grains. Try to limit your intake of refined carbohydrates and be sure to select carbs from the Starches and Breads list and the Vegetables list in this chapter.

4. Limit your intake of saturated fats. Incorporate more unsaturated fats, particularly fish and olive, canola, and flaxseed oils, into your daily diet.

5. Grill, broil, or bake your meats and fish instead of frying them.

6. Take a multivitamin and mineral supplement. Also take calcium if you are not getting at least three servings a day of high-calcium foods, such as milk, yogurt, or calcium-fortified juice. (See chapter 5 for suggestions on supplementation.)

7. Don't skip meals, and try not to go longer than four hours without eating.

Remember that your meal plan is a framework to guide you toward appropriate food selections. While it is okay to deviate from this plan, within reason, remember that you will get the best results by sticking to it as consistently as possible.

Carolyn, a client, discovered the importance of sticking with the food plan when performing a high-intensity exercise program. She says: "Eating properly while you are working out four days a week makes a big difference. A lot of people think that your food choices don't matter that much as long as you're doing the exercises. Yes, you'll still get some benefit. But when you really stick to the diet, the results are amazing. For me, it was seventy percent diet and thirty percent exercise. What you put in your mouth has so much to do with what you are burning and what you are building. If you don't follow the food plan, you're just kidding yourself. You can work out all you want, but you won't get the same results."

Anybody can follow a food program for six weeks. And what's easy about the Lean and Hard Nutritional Plan is that everything is spelled out for you—how often to eat and what to eat. And in the following chapter I even provide you with several delicious sample meal plans for several caloric levels.

Keep in mind that it is all right to allow yourself a treat that you enjoy once or twice a week, simply for pleasure. Good, consistent nutritional habits deserve a reward.

Starches and Breads

Each food listed contains about 15 grams of carbohydrate, 3 grams of protein, a trace of fat, and 80 calories. Whole-grain products are high in fiber and should be included as often as possible.

Cereals, Grains, and Pasta

Bran cereals, dense (such as All-Bran and Fiber One)	⅓ cup
Bran cereals, flaked	¾ cup
Bulgur, cooked	½ cup
Cooked cereals (grits, oatmeal)	½ cup
Grape-Nuts	3 tbsp.
Pasta, cooked	½ cup
Rice, white or brown	⅓ cup
Sushi rolls	4–6 pieces
Wheat germ	3 tbsp.

Dried Beans, Peas, and Lentils

Beans (kidney, white, navy), peas (split, black-eyed), lentils, cooked	⅓ cup
Baked beans	¼ cup
Edamame (steamed, in the pod)	1 cup
Hummus	3 tbsp.

Starchy Vegetables

Corn	½ cup
Green peas	½ cup
Lima beans	½ cup
Potato, baked	1 small
Potato, mashed	½ cup
Squash, winter (acorn, butternut)	1 cup
Yam, sweet potato	⅓ cup

Breads

Bagel, large deli or coffee shop size	¼
Bagel, standard size	½ (1 oz.)
Croutons	1 cup
English muffin	½
Hot dog or hamburger bun	½ (1 oz.)
Pita, 6 inches across (wheat)	½
Plain roll, small	1 (1 oz.)
Rye, pumpernickel, white, and whole-wheat breads	1 slice
Tortilla, 6 inches	1

Crackers and Snacks

Animal crackers	8
Graham crackers	1½ sheets
Melba toast	5 slices
Oyster crackers	24
Popcorn, popped, no fat added	3 cups
Pretzels	¾ oz.
Saltines	6
Triscuits (reduced fat)	4
Triscuit Thin Crisps	8
Wasa Fiber Rye	3 sheets

Starchy Foods Prepared with Fat

Count these starchy foods as one starch/bread unit plus one fat unit. Try to limit your intake of foods from this group, unless they are modified to be lower in fat.

Biscuit, 2½ inches across	1
Corn bread, 2-inch cube	1 (2 oz.)
Cracker, round butter type (e.g., Ritz)	6
French fries, 2–3½ inches long	10 (1½ oz.)
Muffin, small	1
Pancake, 4 inches across	2
Stuffing, bread	¼ cup
Taco shell, 6 inches across	2
Waffle, 4½-inch square	1

Meat and Meat Substitutes

I encourage you to choose more lean and medium-fat meat, poultry (preferably boneless and skinless chicken breasts), and fish for your meal plans. This will help decrease your fat intake, which studies have shown helps to decrease your risk of heart disease. The items from the high-fat group are high in saturated fat, cholesterol, and calories. Therefore, you should limit your choices from this group to three per week. Meat and meat substitutes do not contribute any fiber to your meal plan. Keep the following in mind:

- Each serving contains 7 grams of protein.
- The number of calories and the amount of fat vary, depending on whether the meat product is lean, medium fat, or high fat.
- Two ounces of meat (two meat units) equal 1 small chicken leg or thigh, ½ cup of cottage cheese, or ½ cup of tuna.

- Three ounces of meat (three meat units) equal one medium pork chop, one small burger, ½ whole chicken breast, or one fish fillet about the size of a deck of cards.

Lean Meat and Meat Substitutes

Beef	USDA select or choice grades of lean beef round, sirloin, flank steak, tenderloin, fillet, at least 93 to 96 percent lean ground beef	1 oz.
Pork	Lean pork, ham, tenderloin, Canadian bacon, center-cut pork chops	1 oz.
Veal	All cuts are lean except veal cutlets	1 oz.
Poultry	Skinless and boneless chicken and turkey	1 oz.
Fish	All fresh and frozen fish	1 oz.
	Crab, lobster, shrimp, crawfish, clams	1 oz.
	Oysters	6 medium
	Tuna (canned in water)	¼ cup
Cheese	Cottage cheese (low fat)	¼ cup
	Grated Parmesan	2 tbsp.
	Reduced-calorie cheeses (2 percent cheese)	1 oz.
Other	95 percent fat-free luncheon meat	1½ oz.
	Egg whites	2
	Egg substitute (less than 55 calories)	½ cup

Medium-Fat Meat and Meat Substitutes

Beef	Most beef products: all ground beef, meat loaf, roast (rib, chuck, rump), steak (cubed, T-bone)	1 oz.
Pork	Most pork products: chops, loin roast, cutlets	1 oz.
Veal	Cutlet (ground or cubed, unbreaded)	1 oz.
Poultry	Chicken with skin, domestic duck or goose, ground turkey	1 oz.
Fish	Tuna (canned in oil and drained), salmon (canned)	1 oz.
Cheese	Skim or part skim, such as:	
	Ricotta	¼ cup
	Mozzarella	1 oz.
	Reduced-calorie cheeses (56 to 80 calories per ounce)	1 oz.

Other	Lean luncheon meat	1 oz.
	Egg	1
	Egg substitute (56 to 80 calories per ¼ cup)	½ cup
	Tofu	4 oz.

Vegetables

Vegetables contain 2 to 3 grams of dietary fiber per serving and are a good source of vitamins and minerals. Each serving on this list contains about 5 grams of carbohydrate, 2 grams of protein, and 25 calories. Vegetables that have 100 milligrams or more of sodium per exchange are marked with an asterisk (*). Make fresh and frozen vegetables your first choice because they have more vitamins and less added salt. Rinsing canned vegetables will help to remove much of the salt.

Unless otherwise noted, the serving size for vegetables (one exchange) is ½ cup of cooked vegetables or vegetable juice or 1 cup of raw vegetables.

Artichoke (½ medium)	Mushrooms
Asparagus	Okra
Beans	Onions
Bean sprouts	Pea pods
Broccoli	Peppers
Brussels sprouts	Rutabaga
Cabbage, cooked	Sauerkraut*
Carrots	Spinach, cooked
Cauliflower	Summer squash
Eggplant	Tomatoes
Greens	Turnips
Kohlrabi	Water chestnuts
Leeks	Zucchini, cooked

Starchy vegetables such as corn, peas, and potatoes are found on the starch/bread list. For free vegetables, meaning those that you can eat in abundance, see the free food list on page 51.

Fruits

Each item on the list contains about 15 grams of carbohydrate and 60 calories. Fresh, frozen, and dried fruits have about 2 grams of fiber per exchange. Fruits that have 3 grams or more of fiber per exchange are marked with an asterisk (*). Fruit juices contain very little dietary fiber.

The carbohydrate and calorie content for a fruit exchange is based on the usual serving of the most commonly eaten fruits. Use fresh fruits or frozen or canned fruits without any sugar added. Whole fruit is more filling than fruit juice and may be a better choice for those trying to lose weight.

Unless otherwise noted, the serving size for one fruit exchange is ½ cup of fresh fruit or fruit juice or ¼ cup of dried fruit.

Fresh, Frozen, and Unsweetened, Canned

Apple	1 small, raw
Applesauce (unsweetened)	½ cup
Apricots	4 medium, raw
Apricots (canned)	½ cup or 4 halves
Banana	½, 9 inches long
Blackberries*	¾ cup, raw
Blueberries*	¾ cup, raw
Cantaloupe	⅓ medium
Cherries, raw	12 large
Cherries, canned	½ cup
Figs, raw	2, 2 inches diameter
Fruit cocktail	½ cup, canned
Grapefruit	½ medium
Grapefruit segments	¾ cup
Grapes	15 small
Honeydew melon	½ medium
Kiwi	1 large
Mandarin oranges	¾ cup
Mango	½ cup
Nectarine*	1 small
Orange	1 small
Papaya	1 cup
Peach	1 small or ¾ cup
Peaches	½ cup or 2 halves, canned
Pear	½ large or 1 small
Pears	½ cup or 2 halves, canned
Persimmons	2 medium
Pineapple	¾ cup, raw
Pineapple	⅓ cup, canned
Plums	2, raw

Pomegranate*	½
Raspberries*	1 cup, raw
Strawberries*	1¼ cups, raw, whole
Tangerines*	2 small
Watermelon	1¼ cups, cubed

Dried Fruit

Apples*	4 rings
Apricots*	7 halves
Dates	2½ medium
Figs*	½
Prunes*	3 medium
Raisins	2 tbsp.

Fruit Juice

Apple juice/cider	½ cup
Cranberry juice cocktail	⅓ cup
Grape juice	⅓ cup
Grapefruit juice	½ cup
Orange juice	½ cup
Pineapple juice	½ cup
Prune juice	⅓ cup

Milk

Each serving of milk or milk products on this list contains about 12 grams of carbohydrate and 8 grams of protein. The amount of fat in milk is measured in the percent of butterfat present. Therefore, this list is divided into three categories—skim milk/very-low-fat milk, low-fat milk, and whole milk—based on the amount of fat and calories contained in each serving. One serving (one exchange) of each of these provides calories and nutrients as follows:

	Carbohydrate (grams)	Protein (grams)	Fat (grams)	Calories
Skim/very low fat	12	8	Trace	90
Low fat	12	8	5	120
Whole	12	8	8	150

Milk is the body's main source of calcium, the mineral needed for growth and bone repair. Yogurt is also a good source of calcium (you can add life to plain yogurt by adding one of your fruit exchanges to it). However, since each brand of yogurt may have a different amount of fat, always read the label to find out the fat and calorie content. The same goes for dry or powdered milk products.

Milk can also be added to cereal and to other foods. Many tasty dishes such as sugar-free pudding are made with milk.

Skim and Very-Low-Fat Milk

Skim milk	1 cup
½ percent milk	1 cup
1 percent milk	1 cup
Low-fat buttermilk	1 cup
Evaporated skim milk	½ cup
Dry nonfat milk	½ cup
Plain nonfat yogurt	8 oz.

Low-Fat Milk

2 percent milk	1 cup
Plain low-fat yogurt (with added nonfat milk solids)	8 oz.

Whole Milk

The whole milk group has much more fat per serving than the skim and low-fat groups. Since whole milk has more than 3¼ percent butter, limit your exchanges to the lower-fat milks as much as possible.

Whole milk	1 cup
Evaporated whole milk	½ cup
Whole plain yogurt	8 oz.

Fats

Each serving on the fat list contains about 5 grams of fat and 45 calories. While these foods are mostly fat, some exchanges also contain a small amount of protein. Since all fats are high in calories, your intake of these foods should be carefully measured. While I have divided the fats list into unsaturated fats, saturated fats, and trans-fatty acids, your first choice should always be unsaturated fats whenever possible.

Remember to read labels because the sodium content of these foods varies widely. You will notice symbols on some foods in the exchange groups. Foods that have 400 milligrams or more of sodium if two or more exchanges are eaten are marked with an asterisk (*). It's a good idea to limit your intake of high-salt foods, especially if you have high blood pressure.

Unsaturated Fats

Avocado	⅛ medium
Margarine	1 tsp.
Margarine, low fat*	1 tbsp.
Mayonnaise	1 tsp.
Mayonnaise (reduced calorie)*	1 tbsp.
Nuts and Seeds	
Almonds, dry roasted	6 whole
Cashews, dry roasted	1 tbsp.
Peanuts	20 small or 10 large
Pecans	2 whole
Walnuts	2 whole
Other nuts	1 tbsp.
Pine nuts, sunflower seeds (without shells)	1 tbsp.
Pumpkin seeds	2 tsp.
Oil (corn, cottonseed, safflower, olive, peanut, canola)	1 tsp.
Olives*	10 small or 5 large
Salad dressing, mayonnaise type	1 tsp.
Salad dressing, mayonnaise type, reduced calorie	1 tbsp.
Salad dressing (oil varieties)*	1 tbsp.
Salad dressing, low calorie†	2 tbsp.

† Two tablespoons of low-calorie salad dressing is a free food

Saturated Fats

Bacon*	1 slice
Butter	1 tsp.
Coconut, shredded	½ oz.
Coffee creamer, liquid	2 tbsp.
Coffee creamer, powder	4 tsp.
Cream (heavy, whipping)	1 tbsp.
Cream (light, coffee, table)	2 tbsp.
Cream, sour	2 tbsp.

Cream cheese	1 tbsp.
Salt pork*	¼ oz.

Trans-Fatty Acids

Regular intake of this type of fat increases your risk of heart disease by raising your LDL (bad) cholesterol. To determine whether a food product contains trans-fatty acids, look for the words "partially hydrogenated" on the ingredient list.

The following is a list of foods that are high in trans-fatty acids:

Baked goods

Cookies

Margarine

Peanut butter, processed (not natural)

Potato chips

Free Foods

A free food is any food or drink that contains less than 20 calories per serving. You may eat two or three servings per day of free foods that have a specified serving size; you can eat as much as you want of those that have no specified serving size. Be sure to spread your free food choices throughout the day. Foods that have 100 milligrams or more of sodium per exchange are marked with an asterisk (*). Foods that have 3 grams or more of fiber per exchange are marked with a dagger (†).

Drinks

Bouillon* or broth without fat

Bouillon, low-sodium

Carbonated drinks, sugar free

Carbonated water

Club soda

Cocoa powder, unsweetened (1 tbsp.)

Coffee/tea

Drink mixes, sugar free

Tonic water, sugar free

Fruit

Cranberries, unsweetened (½ cup)

Rhubarb, unsweetened (½ cup)

Vegetables (raw, 1 cup)

Cabbage

Celery

Chinese cabbage[†]

Cucumber

Green onion

Hot peppers

Mushrooms

Radishes

Zucchini[†]

Salad Greens

Endive

Escarole

Lettuce

Romaine

Spinach

Sweets Substitutes

Candy, hard, sugar free

Gelatin, sugar free

Gum, sugar free

Jam/jelly, sugar free (less than 20 calories per 2 tsp.)

Pancake syrup, sugar free (1–2 tbsp.)

Sugar substitutes (saccharin, aspartame)

Whipped topping

Condiments

Horseradish

Ketchup (1 tbsp.)

Mustard

Pickles, dill, unsweetened

Salad dressing, low calorie (2 tbsp.)

Taco sauce

Vinegar

Seasonings

Seasonings can add zest to your meals. The only thing to watch out for is how much sodium a particular seasoning contains. Read the labels and choose those that do not contain sodium or salt. Foods that have 100 milligrams or more of sodium per exchange are marked with an asterisk (*).

Basil (fresh)
Celery seeds
Chili powder
Chives
Cinnamon
Curry
Dill
Garlic
Garlic powder
Herbs
Hot pepper sauce
Lemon
Lemon juice
Lemon pepper
Lime
Lime juice
Mint
Onion powder
Paprika
Oregano
Pepper
Pimiento
Soy sauce*
Soy sauce, low sodium
Spices
Wine, used in cooking
Worcestershire sauce

Flavoring Extracts
Almond
Peppermint

Vanilla

Walnut

Fats

Nonstick pan spray

Now that you've had a chance to familiarize yourself with how the food exchange lists and free foods work, you can find some sample daily menus in the following chapter.

5

Lean and Hard Meal Plans for High Performance

Following are several high-performance meal plans developed by the sports nutritionist Tavis Piattoly, director of Sports Performance at Elmwood Fitness Center. Keep in mind that your daily caloric needs depend upon your weight and energy requirements, especially if you are a very large person with a high weight. To cover all contingencies, I have included high-intensity training meal plans up to 5,000 calories per day. We have divided them into six caloric spreads: 2,500 calories, 3,000 calories, 3,500 calories, 4,000 calories, 4,500 calories, and 5,000 calories. These delicious main meals and snacks should serve as guidelines to help you eat well to support your HIT workout.

Here are a few general points:

- Unless otherwise indicated, the ideal beverage of choice for each meal or snack should be water or unsweetened tea.
- All poultry should be boneless and skinless breasts.
- For drinks containing whey protein, select a brand that contains only 2 grams of carbs for every 10 grams of protein.

Meal Plans for the 2,500-Calorie Program

The meal plans below, divided into options for breakfast, lunch, dinner, and snacks, are designed so that if you eat three meals and two snacks per day, you will be ingesting 2,500 calories.

Breakfast Options

1 cup of cooked oatmeal with 1 tbsp. of ground flaxseed (optional), or stir in 20 g of whey protein powder.
2–3 low-fat and/or vegetarian sausage patties (try Healthy Choice, Morningstar Farms, or Boca varieties).
8 oz. of 100 percent juice.
1 container of light yogurt.

1 carton of Egg Beaters, scrambled, with 1 thin slice each of cheddar cheese and lean ham, rolled into 2 small whole-wheat tortillas (look for at least 3 g of fiber; we like La Tortilla Factory, with 8–9 g of fiber per tortilla).
12 oz. of skim or soy milk (or 1 container of light yogurt) or 8–12 oz. of juice.

2 breakfast burritos, using small (1-oz.) whole-wheat tortillas with 3 egg whites plus 1 yolk, 2 tbsp. of salsa (optional), and ¼ cup of diced onions and green peppers.
8 oz. of skim or soy milk (or add 1 oz. of cheese to the burritos).
1 piece of fresh fruit.

2 slices of 100 percent whole-grain bread (at least 3 g of fiber per slice).
1 whole egg plus 3 egg whites, prepared any way you like.
1 cup of light applesauce (try Lucky Leaf).
8 oz. of 100 percent juice.

2 whole-grain waffles such as Kashi or Van's 7-grain frozen waffles, or made from a whole-wheat baking mix such as Hodgson Mill, topped with 1 tbsp. of peanut butter (preferably natural).
8 oz. of skim or soy milk.
1 container of light yogurt or 1 piece of fresh fruit.

1½ cups of whole-wheat pasta (yes, it can be a great breakfast, for all you pasta lovers!) drizzled with 1 tsp. of olive oil with 2 oz. of lean protein tossed in—such as chicken or shrimp (you can also sprinkle ¼ cup of light mozzarella cheese on top).
12 oz. of 100 percent juice.

1 grab-and-go sandwich: 2 slices of whole-grain bread, 3 slices of turkey, and a thin slice of cheese—throw it together, fold it over, and you've got a great breakfast for the road.
1 piece of fresh fruit.
12 oz. of 100 percent juice or low-fat milk.

protein shake: mix 20 g of whey protein powder (should contain no more than 4 g of carbohydrate per 20 g) with 12 oz. of skim or soy milk, 1–2 tbsp. of ground flaxseed, and 1 cup of fresh or frozen berries (no sugar added). Add ice and blend.

Snack Options

Anytime you are going more than four hours between meals, you should make sure that you have a snack to boost your metabolism and stabilize insulin levels. Below are some suggestions for midmorning and midafternoon snacks.

1 small red apple with 1 tbsp. of almond butter on 1 slice of whole-grain bread.

8 whole-grain crackers (e.g., woven wheat crackers) topped with sliced mozzarella (approximately 1 oz.) and 1 piece of fresh fruit.

trail mix: 2 tbsp. of raisins with 10–12 mixed nuts and ½ cup of dried fruit.

½ cup of low-fat cottage cheese with 1 cup of fresh berries and 1 container of light yogurt.

12–15 low-fat chips (e.g., Sun Chips, which are high in fiber) with 3 tbsp. of bean dip or hummus and a 2–3 oz. chicken breast.

2 whole-wheat tortillas (try La Tortilla Factory) topped with 3 tbsp. of low-fat shredded cheddar, melted. Roll up and dip into salsa.

½ cup of Kashi GOLEAN Crunch! cereal mixed with 1 container of light yogurt.

at a smoothie store or a gym smoothie bar: Myoplex Lite blended with 1 percent milk (my favorite flavor: Cappuccino Ice).

protein shake: mix 20 g whey protein powder (should contain no more than 4 g of carbohydrate per 20 g) with 4 oz. of water and 4 oz. of skim or soy milk and 1 tbsp. of ground flaxseed (optional). Add ice and blend.

2 squares of dark chocolate (look for at least 70 percent cocoa) with 10–12 nuts (try almonds or walnuts for added omega-3 fatty acids).

Lunch Options

5 oz. of seared tuna on a large bed of mixed greens topped with 1 tbsp. of chopped walnuts and drizzled with red wine vinaigrette.
1 small sweet potato (4 oz.) topped with fresh ground cinnamon and 1 tsp. of Brummel and Brown butter.

tuna, chicken, or salmon salad: mix a 5-oz. can with 1 tbsp. of real mayonnaise, pepper, a splash of lemon juice, and 1 tsp. of olive oil. Serve over a bed of romaine, with 10 whole-grain crackers (try Triscuits or 100 percent whole-wheat stone-ground crackers).

5-oz. chicken breast brushed lightly with barbecue sauce.
1 small sweet potato (4 oz.); add ground cinnamon and 2 tsp. of butter (try Brummel and Brown).
1–2 cups of green beans, sautéed with garlic and 1 tsp. of olive oil.

1 cup of whole-wheat pasta topped with red sauce and 5 oz. of extralean ground turkey breast (try Honeysuckle).
1 cup of steamed broccoli (top with ¼ cup of Parmesan cheese).
spinach salad drizzled with light Italian dressing.

grilled chicken fajitas: use 2 small whole-wheat tortillas and 4 oz. of chicken breast. Add ¼ cup of light cheese, ¼ cup of salsa, and ¼ cup of diced onions and green peppers (optional).

5 oz. extralean turkey burger (try Honeysuckle extralean ground turkey) on a wheat bun.
side salad: a bed of mixed romaine and spinach leaves with light Italian dressing; add any vegetables you like.

5 oz. of grilled fish with 1 cup of lentils and broiled tomatoes (slice 1 whole tomato) topped with fresh mozzarella cheese (1 oz).

5 oz. of shrimp or crawfish, stir-fried with mushrooms, spinach, onions, and minced garlic in 1 tsp. of olive oil and a splash of soy sauce. Serve over ¾ cup of brown rice or 1 cup of whole-wheat pasta.
1 cup of grilled or sautéed asparagus.

1 whole-wheat tortilla wrap (try La Tortilla Factory) with 4 oz. of turkey or chicken (for turkey, try Honeysuckle's extralean turkey breast), 1 thin deli slice of cheese, and 1 cup of cooked vegetables (onions, green peppers, tomatoes).
steamed broccoli and cauliflower.

pita pocket sandwich: stuff 5 oz. of your favorite lean protein (turkey, chicken, tuna, or extralean ground beef) into 1 whole-wheat pita (2 pockets). Add fresh spinach leaves, sliced red peppers, and a drizzle of light vinaigrette dressing.

protein shake: mix 20 g of whey protein powder (should contain no more than 4 g of carbohydrate per 20 g) with 12 oz. of skim or soy milk, 1–2 tbsp. of ground flaxseed, 2 tbsp. of peanut butter, and 1 cup of fresh or frozen berries (no sugar added). Add ice and blend.

Dinner Options

5 oz. of grilled tuna or salmon with portobello mushrooms and red peppers, grilled or roasted, with 1 tsp. olive oil and seasonings. Serve over ¾ cup of brown rice.

shrimp-veggie lo-mein: 6 oz. of grilled shrimp (grill in a wok or a pan with about 2 tsp. of olive oil). Serve over 1 cup of whole-wheat pasta (long; try Barilla or Hodgson Mill) and mixed sautéed vegetables (broccoli, zucchini, squash, tomatoes, and onions). You can add these to the wok once the shrimp is cooked.

meat loaf (5 oz.); use extralean ground beef (96 percent lean).
1 small baked potato (4 oz); add ¼ cup of low-fat shredded cheese and 1 tsp. of Brummel and Brown butter if you like.
mixed green salad tossed with 1 tbsp. of light vinaigrette dressing.

2 shrimp and chicken kabobs, made with any vegetables you like (mushrooms, onions, and peppers work well).
1 small sweet potato (4 oz); add cinnamon and 2 tsp. of Brummel and Brown butter.
grilled or sautéed vegetables of choice.

turkey breast fillet (5 oz.)
1 small baked potato (4 oz.); add 2 tsp. of Brummel and Brown butter and ⅓ cup of low-fat cheddar cheese.
1–2 cups of steamed broccoli with ¼ cup of Parmesan cheese.

pork tenderloin medallions (4 oz.).
1 cup of whole-wheat fettuccini noodles (add 2 tbsp. of minced garlic, 2 tsp. of olive oil, and ¼ cup of Parmesan cheese).
1–2 cups of asparagus, steamed with a splash each of lemon juice and balsamic vinegar.

protein shake: mix 20 g of whey protein powder (should contain no more than 4 g of carbohydrates per 20 g) with 12 oz. of skim or soy milk, 1–2 tbsp. of ground flaxseed, 1 tbsp. of peanut butter, and 1 cup of fresh or frozen berries (no sugar added). Add ice and blend.

Meal Plans for the 3,000-Calorie Program

The meal plans below, divided into options for breakfast, lunch, dinner, and snacks, are designed so that if you eat three meals and two snacks per day, you will be ingesting 3,000 calories.

Breakfast Options

1 cup of cooked oatmeal with 1 tbsp. of ground flaxseed (optional), or stir in 20 g of whey protein powder.

2–3 low-fat and/or vegetarian sausage patties (try Healthy Choice, Morningstar Farms, or Boca varieties).

12 oz. of 100 percent juice.

1 container of light yogurt.

1 carton of Egg Beaters, scrambled, with 1 thin slice each of cheddar cheese and lean ham, rolled into 2 small whole-wheat tortillas (look for at least 3 g of fiber; we like La Tortilla Factory, with 8–9 g of fiber per tortilla).

12 oz. of skim or soy milk (or 1 container of light yogurt) or 8–12 oz. of juice.

1 piece of fresh fruit.

2 breakfast burritos, using small (1-oz.) whole-wheat tortillas (try La Tortilla Factory) with 4 egg whites plus 1 yolk, 2 tbsp. of salsa (optional), ¼ cup of low-fat cheese, and ¼ cup of diced onions and green peppers.

12 oz. of skim or soy milk (or add 1 oz. of cheese to the burritos).

1 medium piece of fresh fruit (e.g., medium apple or pear, 6 oz.).

2 slices of 100 percent whole-grain bread (at least 3 g of fiber per slice).

1 whole egg plus 4 egg whites, prepared any way you like.

1 cup of light applesauce (try Lucky Leaf).

12 oz. of 100 percent juice.

2 whole-grain waffles such as Kashi or Van's 7-grain frozen waffles, or made from a whole-wheat baking mix such as Hodgson Mill, each topped with 1 tbsp. of peanut butter (preferably natural).

12 oz. of skim or soy milk.

1 container of light yogurt or 1 piece of fresh fruit.

1½ cups of whole-wheat pasta (yes, it can be a great breakfast, for all you pasta lovers!) drizzled with 1 tsp. of olive oil with 4 oz. of lean protein tossed in—such as chicken or shrimp (you can also sprinkle ¼ cup of light mozzarella cheese on top).

12 oz. of 100 percent juice.

grab-and-go sandwich: 2 slices of whole-grain bread, 4 slices of turkey, and a thin slice of cheese—throw it together, fold it over, and you've got a great breakfast for the road.

1 piece of fresh fruit.

12 oz. of 100 percent juice or low-fat milk.

protein shake: mix 30 g of whey protein powder (should contain no more than 4 g of carbohydrates per 20 g) with 12 oz. of skim or soy milk, 1–2 tbsp. of ground flaxseed, and 1 cup of fresh or frozen berries (no sugar added). Add ice and blend.

Snack Options

Anytime you are going more than four hours between meals, you should make sure that you have a snack to boost your metabolism and stabilize insulin levels. Below are some suggestions for midmorning and midafternoon snacks.

1 medium red apple with 1 tbsp. of almond butter on 1 slice of whole-grain bread.

10 whole-grain crackers (e.g., woven wheat crackers) topped with sliced mozzarella (approximately 1 oz.) and 1 piece of fresh fruit.

trail mix: 3 tbsp. of raisins with 10–12 mixed nuts and 1 cup of dried fruit.

1 cup of low-fat cottage cheese with 1½ cups of fresh berries and 1 container of light yogurt.

15 low-fat chips (e.g., Sun Chips, which are high in fiber) with 3 tbsp. of bean dip or hummus and a 4 oz. chicken breast.

2 whole-wheat tortillas (try La Tortilla Factory) topped with 3 tbsp. of low-fat shredded cheddar, melted. Roll up and dip into salsa.

1 cup of Kashi GOLEAN Crunch! cereal mixed with 1 container of light yogurt.

at a smoothie store or a gym smoothie bar: Myoplex Lite blended with 1 percent milk (my favorite flavor: Cappuccino Ice).

protein shake: mix 30 g of whey protein (powder should contain no more than 4 g of carbohydrates per 20 g) with 8 oz. of skim or soy milk and 1 tbsp. of ground flaxseed (optional). Add ice and blend.

2 squares of dark chocolate (look for at least 70 percent cocoa) with 10–12 nuts (try almonds or walnuts for added omega-3 fatty acids).

Lunch Options

6–8 oz. of seared tuna on a large bed of mixed greens topped with 1 tbsp. of chopped walnuts and drizzled with red wine vinaigrette.
1 medium sweet potato (6–8 oz.) topped with fresh ground cinnamon and 1 tsp. of Brummel and Brown butter.

tuna, chicken, or salmon salad: mix a 6-oz. can with 1 tbsp. of real mayonnaise, pepper, a splash of lemon juice, and 1 tsp. of olive oil. Serve over a bed of romaine, with 12 whole-grain crackers (try Triscuits or 100 percent whole-wheat stone-ground crackers).

6-oz. chicken breast brushed lightly with barbecue sauce.
1 medium sweet potato (6-8 oz.); add ground cinnamon and 1 tbsp. of butter (try
Brummel and Brown).
1–2 cups of green beans, sautéed with garlic and 2 tsp. of olive oil.

1½ cups of whole-wheat pasta topped with red sauce and 6 oz. of extralean ground
turkey breast (try Honeysuckle).
2 cups of steamed broccoli (top with ¼ cup of Parmesan cheese).
spinach salad drizzled with light Italian dressing.

grilled chicken fajitas: use 2–3 small whole-wheat tortillas (try La Tortilla Factory) and
6 oz. of chicken breast. Add ½ cup of brown rice, ¼ cup of light cheese, ¼–½ cup
of salsa, and ¼ cup of diced onions and green peppers (optional).

6-oz. extralean turkey burger (try Honeysuckle extralean ground turkey) on a wheat
bun.
side salad: bed of mixed romaine and spinach leaves with light Italian dressing; add
any vegetables you like.

6 oz. of grilled fish with 1½ cups of lentils and broiled tomatoes (slice 1 whole
tomato) topped with fresh mozzarella cheese (1 oz.).

6 oz. of shrimp or crawfish stir-fried with mushrooms, spinach, onions, and minced
garlic in 2 tsp. of olive oil and a splash of soy sauce. Serve over ¾ cup of brown rice
or 1 cup of whole-wheat pasta.
2 cups of grilled or sautéed asparagus.

2 whole-wheat tortilla wraps (try La Tortilla Factory) with 6 oz. of turkey or chicken
(for turkey, try Honeysuckle extralean turkey breast), 1 thin deli slice of cheese, and
cooked vegetables (onions, green peppers, tomatoes).
steamed broccoli and cauliflower.

pita pocket sandwich: stuff 6 oz. of your favorite lean protein (turkey, chicken, tuna,
or extralean ground beef) into 1 whole-wheat pita (2 pockets). Add fresh spinach
leaves, sliced red peppers, and a drizzle of light vinaigrette dressing.

protein shake: mix 30 g of whey protein powder (should contain no more than 4 g of
carbohydrates per 20 g) with 12 oz. of skim or soy milk, 2 tbsp. of ground flaxseed,
2 tbsp. of peanut butter, and 1 cup of fresh or frozen berries (no sugar added). Add
ice and blend.

Dinner Options

6 oz. of grilled tuna or salmon with portobello mushrooms and red peppers, grilled
or roasted, with 2 tsp. of olive oil and seasonings. Serve over ¾ cup of brown
rice.

shrimp-veggie lo-mein: 6 oz. of grilled shrimp (grill in a wok or a pan with about 2 tsp. of olive oil). Serve over 1½ cups of whole-wheat pasta (long; try Barilla or Hodgson Mill) and mixed sautéed vegetables (broccoli, zucchini, squash, tomatoes, and onions). You can add these to the wok once the shrimp is cooked.

meat loaf (6 oz.); use extralean ground beef (96 percent lean).
1 medium baked potato (6 oz.); add ¼ cup of low-fat shredded cheese and 2 tsp. of Brummel and Brown butter.
mixed green salad tossed with 1 tbsp. of light vinaigrette dressing.

3 shrimp and chicken kabobs, made with any vegetables you like (mushrooms, onions and peppers work well).
1 medium sweet potato (6 oz.); add cinnamon and 2 tsp. of Brummel and Brown butter.
grilled or sautéed vegetables of choice.

turkey breast fillet (6 oz.)
1 medium baked potato (6 oz.); add 2 tsp. of Brummel and Brown butter and ⅓ cup of low-fat cheddar cheese.
2 cups of steamed broccoli with ¼ cup of Parmesan cheese.

pork tenderloin medallions (6 oz.)
1½ cups of whole-wheat fettuccini noodles (add 2 tbsp. of minced garlic, 2 tsp. of olive oil, and ¼ cup of Parmesan cheese).
2 cups of asparagus, steamed with a splash each of lemon juice and balsamic vinegar.

protein shake: mix 30 g of whey protein powder (should contain no more than 4 g of carbohydrates) with 12 oz. of skim or soy milk, 1–2 tbsp. of ground flaxseed, 2 tbsp. of peanut butter, and 1 cup of fresh or frozen berries (no sugar added). Add ice and blend.

Meal Plans for the 3,500 Calorie Program

The meal plans below, divided into options for breakfast, lunch, dinner, and snacks, are designed so that if you eat three meals and two snacks per day, you will be ingesting 3,500 calories.

Breakfast Options

1 cup of cooked oatmeal with 1 tbsp. of ground flaxseed (optional), or stir in 30 g of whey protein powder.
3 low-fat and/or vegetarian sausage patties (try Healthy Choice, Morningstar Farms, or Boca varieties).
16 oz. of 100 percent juice.
1 container of light yogurt.

1 carton of Egg Beaters, scrambled, with 2 thin slices each of cheddar cheese and lean ham, rolled into 2 small whole-wheat tortillas (look for at least 3 g of fiber; we like La Tortilla Factory, with 8–9 g of fiber per tortilla).
16 oz. of skim or soy milk (or 1 container of light yogurt) or 8–12 oz. of juice.
1 piece of fresh fruit.

2 breakfast burritos, using small (1-oz.) whole-wheat tortillas with 5 egg whites plus 1 yolk, 2 tbsp. of salsa (optional), ⅓ cup of low-fat cheese, and ¼ cup of diced onions and green peppers.
12 oz. of skim or soy milk (or add 1 oz. of cheese to the burritos).
1 large piece of fresh fruit (e.g., an apple or a pear, 8 oz.).

3 slices of 100 percent whole-grain bread (at least 3 g of fiber per slice).
1 whole egg plus 5 egg whites, prepared any way you like.
1 cup of light applesauce (try Lucky Leaf).
16 oz. of 100 percent juice.

2 whole-grain waffles such as Kashi or Van's 7-grain frozen waffles, or made from a whole-wheat baking mix such as Hodgson Mill, topped with 1 tbsp. of peanut butter (preferably natural).
16 oz. of skim or soy milk.
1 container of light yogurt or 1 piece of fresh fruit.

2 cups of whole-wheat pasta (yes, it can be a great breakfast, for all you pasta lovers!) drizzled with 1 tsp. of olive oil with 5–6 oz. of lean protein tossed in—such as chicken or shrimp (you can also sprinkle ¼ cup of light mozzarella cheese on top).
16 oz. of 100 percent juice.

grab-and-go sandwich: 2 slices of whole-grain bread, 5 slices of turkey, and a thin slice of cheese—throw it together, fold it over, and you've got a great breakfast for the road.
1 piece of fresh fruit.
16 oz. of 100 percent juice or low-fat milk.

protein shake: mix 40 g of whey protein powder (should contain no more than 4 g of carbohydrates per 20 g) with 12 oz. of skim or soy milk, 2 tbsp. of peanut butter, 1–2 tbsp. of ground flaxseed, and 1 cup of fresh or frozen berries (no sugar added). Add ice and blend.

Snack Options

Anytime you are going more than four hours between meals, you should make sure that you have a snack to boost your metabolism and stabilize insulin levels. Below are some suggestions for midmorning and midafternoon snacks.

1 large red apple with 1 tbsp. of almond butter on 1–2 slices of whole-grain bread.

15 whole-grain crackers (e.g., woven wheat crackers) topped with sliced mozzarella (approximately 1 oz.) and 1 piece of fresh fruit.

trail mix: 3 tbsp. raisins with 10–12 mixed nuts and 1 cup of dried fruit.

1 cup of low-fat cottage cheese with 2 cups of fresh berries and 1 container of light yogurt.

15 low-fat chips (e.g., Sun Chips, which are high in fiber) with 3–4 tbsp. of bean dip or hummus and a 4-oz. chicken breast.

2 whole-wheat tortillas (try La Tortilla Factory) topped with 3 tbsp. of low-fat shredded cheddar, melted, and 3 oz. of grilled chicken. Roll up and dip into salsa.

1½ cups of Kashi GOLEAN Crunch! cereal mixed with 1 container of light yogurt.

at a smoothie store or a gym smoothie bar: Myoplex Deluxe blended with 1 percent milk (my favorite flavor: Cappuccino Ice).

protein shake: mix 40 g whey protein powder (should contain no more than 4 g of carbohydrate per 20 g) with 8 oz. of skim or soy milk and 1 tbsp. of ground flaxseed (optional). Add ice and blend.

2 squares of dark chocolate (look for at least 70 percent cocoa) with 10–12 nuts (try almonds or walnuts for added omega-3 fatty acids).

Lunch Options

8 oz. of seared tuna on a large bed of mixed greens topped with 1 tbsp. of chopped walnuts and drizzled with red wine vinaigrette.
1 large sweet potato (8 oz.) topped with fresh ground cinnamon and 2 tsp. of Brummel and Brown butter.

tuna, chicken, or salmon salad: mix an 8-oz. can with 1 tbsp. of real mayonnaise, pepper, a splash of lemon juice, and 1 tsp. of olive oil. Serve over a bed of romaine, with 15 whole-grain crackers (try Triscuits or 100 percent whole-wheat stone-ground crackers) or 2 slices of whole-wheat bread.

8-oz. chicken breast brushed lightly with barbecue sauce.
1 medium sweet potato (8 oz.); add ground cinnamon and 1 tbsp. of butter (try Brummel and Brown).
2 cups of green beans, sautéed with garlic and 1 tbsp. of olive oil.

2 cups of whole-wheat pasta topped with red sauce and 8 oz. of extralean ground turkey breast (try Honeysuckle).
2 cups of steamed broccoli (top with ¼ cup of Parmesan cheese).
spinach salad drizzled with light Italian dressing.

grilled chicken fajitas: use 3 small whole-wheat tortillas (try La Tortilla Factory) and 8 oz. of chicken breast. Add ½ cup of brown rice, ¼ cup of light cheese, ¼–½ cup of salsa, and ¼ cup of diced onions and green peppers (optional).

8-oz. extralean turkey burger (try Honeysuckle extralean ground turkey) on a wheat bun.
side salad: a bed of mixed romaine and spinach leaves with light Italian dressing; add any vegetables you like.

8 oz. of grilled fish with 2 cups of lentils and broiled tomatoes (slice 1 whole tomato) topped with fresh mozzarella cheese (1 oz.).

8 oz. of shrimp or crawfish, stir-fried with mushrooms, spinach, onions, and minced garlic in 2 tsp. of olive oil and a splash of soy sauce. Serve over 1 cup of brown rice or 1 cup of whole-wheat pasta.
2 cups of grilled or sautéed asparagus.

2–3 whole-wheat tortilla wraps (try La Tortilla Factory) with 8 oz. of turkey or chicken, (for turkey, try Honeysuckle's extralean turkey breast), one thin deli slice of cheese, and cooked vegetables (onions, green peppers, tomatoes).
steamed broccoli and cauliflower.

pita pocket sandwich: stuff 8 oz. of your favorite lean protein (turkey, chicken, tuna, or extralean ground beef) into 1–2 whole-wheat pitas (3–4 pockets = 2 pitas). Add fresh spinach leaves, sliced red peppers, and a drizzle of light vinaigrette dressing.

protein shake: mix 40 g of whey protein powder (should contain no more than 4 g of carbohydrates per 20 g) with 12 oz. of skim or soy milk, 2 tbsp. of ground flaxseed, 2 tbsp. of peanut butter, and 1 cup of fresh or frozen berries (no sugar added). Add ice and blend.

Dinner Options

8 oz. of grilled tuna or salmon with portobello mushrooms and red peppers, grilled or roasted, with 2 tsp. of olive oil and seasonings. Serve over ¾ cup of brown rice.

shrimp-veggie lo-mein: 8 oz. of grilled shrimp (grill in a wok or a pan with about 2 tsp. of olive oil). Serve over 2 cups of whole wheat-pasta (long; try Barilla or Hodgson Mill) and mixed sautéed vegetables (broccoli, zucchini, squash, tomatoes, and onions). You can add these to the wok once the shrimp is cooked.

meat loaf (8 oz.); use extralean ground beef (96 percent lean).
1 large baked potato (8 oz); add ¼ cup of low-fat shredded cheese and 2 tsp. of Brummel and Brown butter if you like.
mixed green salad tossed with 1 tbsp. of light vinaigrette dressing.

4 shrimp and chicken kabobs, made with any vegetables you like (mushrooms, onions, and peppers work well).

1 large sweet potato (8 oz); add cinnamon and 2 tsp. of Brummel and Brown butter.

grilled or sautéed vegetables of choice.

turkey breast fillet (8 oz.)

1 large baked potato (8 oz.); add 2 tsp. of Brummel and Brown butter and ⅓ cup of low-fat cheddar cheese.

2 cups of steamed broccoli with ¼ cup of Parmesan cheese.

pork tenderloin medallions (8 oz.)

2 cups of whole-wheat fettuccini noodles (add 2 tbsp. of minced garlic, 1 tbsp. of olive oil, and ¼ cup of Parmesan cheese).

2 cups of asparagus, steamed with a splash each of lemon juice and balsamic vinegar.

protein shake: mix 40 g of whey protein powder (should contain no more than 4 g of carbohydrates per 20 g) with 12 oz. of skim or soy milk, 1–2 tbsp. of ground flaxseed, 2 tbsp. of peanut butter, and 1 cup of fresh or frozen berries (no sugar added). Add ice and blend.

Meal Plans for the 4,000-Calorie Program

The meal plans below, divided into options for breakfast, lunch, dinner, and snacks, are designed so that if you eat three meals and two snacks per day, you will be ingesting 4,000 calories.

Breakfast Options

1½ cups of cooked oatmeal with 1 tbsp. of ground flaxseed (optional), or stir in 30 g of whey protein powder.

3 low-fat and/or vegetarian sausage patties (try Healthy Choice, Morningstar Farms, or Boca varieties).

16 oz. of 100 percent juice.

1 carton of Egg Beaters, scrambled, with 2 thin slices of lean ham, rolled into 2 small whole-wheat tortillas (look for at least 3 g of fiber; we like La Tortilla Factory, with 8–9 g of fiber per tortilla).

12 oz. of skim or soy milk (or 1 container of light yogurt) or 8–12 oz. of juice.

2 breakfast burritos, using small (1-oz.) whole-wheat tortillas (try La Tortilla Factory) with 5 egg whites plus 1 yolk), 2 tbsp. of salsa (optional), ⅓ cup of low-fat cheese, and ¼ cup diced of onions and green peppers.

12 oz. of skim or soy milk (or add 1 oz. of cheese to the burritos).

1 large piece of fresh fruit (an apple or a pear, 8 oz.).

3 slices of 100 percent whole-grain bread (at least 3 g of fiber per slice).
1 whole egg plus 5 egg whites, prepared any way you like.
1 cup of applesauce (sweetened).
16 oz. of 100 percent juice.

2 whole-grain waffles such as Kashi or Van's 7-grain frozen waffles, or made from a
    whole-wheat baking mix such as Hodgson Mill, topped with 1½ tbsp. of peanut but-
    ter (preferably natural).
16 oz. of skim or soy milk.
1 container of light yogurt or 1 piece of fresh fruit.

1½ cups of whole-wheat pasta (yes, it can be a great breakfast, for all you pasta
    lovers!) drizzled with 1 tsp. of olive oil with 5 oz. of lean protein tossed in—such as
    chicken or shrimp (you can also sprinkle ¼ cup of light mozzarella cheese on top).
12 oz. of 100 percent juice.

grab-and-go sandwich: 2 slices of whole-grain bread, 5 slices of turkey, and a thin slice of
    cheese—throw it together, fold it over, and you've got a great breakfast for the road.
1 piece of fresh fruit.
16 oz. of 100 percent juice or low-fat milk.

protein shake: mix 40 g of whey protein powder (should contain no more than 4 g of
    carbohydrates per 20 g) with 12 oz. of skim or soy milk, 2 tbsp. of peanut butter,
    1–2 tbsp. of ground flaxseed, and 1 cup of fresh or frozen berries (no sugar added).
    Add ice and blend.

Snack Options

Anytime you are going more than four hours between meals, you should make
sure that you have a snack to boost your metabolism and stabilize insulin levels.
Below are some suggestions for midmorning and midafternoon snacks.

1 large red apple with 1½ tbsp. of almond butter on 2 slices of whole-grain bread.

12 whole-grain crackers (e.g., woven wheat crackers) topped with sliced mozzarella
    (approximately 1 oz.) and 1 piece of fresh fruit.

trail mix: small box of raisins with 10–12 mixed nuts and ½ cup of dried fruit.

1 cup of low-fat cottage cheese with 2 cups of fresh berries and ½ cup of light yogurt.

15 low-fat chips (e.g., Sun Chips, which are high in fiber) with 3 tbsp. of bean dip or
    hummus and a 3-oz. chicken breast.

1 whole-wheat tortilla (try La Tortilla Factory) topped with 2 tbsp. of low-fat shredded
    cheddar, melted, and 3 oz. of grilled chicken. Roll up and dip into salsa.

1½ cups of Kashi GOLEAN Crunch! cereal mixed with 1 container of light yogurt.

at a smoothie store or a gym smoothie bar: Myoplex Deluxe blended with 1 percent milk (my favorite flavor: Cappuccino Ice).

protein shake: mix 40 g of whey protein powder (should contain no more than 4 g of carbohydrate per 20 g) with 8 oz. of skim or soy milk and 1 tbsp. of ground flaxseed (optional). Add ice and blend.

2 squares of dark chocolate (look for at least 70 percent cocoa) with 10–12 nuts (try almonds or walnuts for added omega 3-fatty acids) and 1 piece of fresh fruit.

Lunch Options

8 oz. of seared tuna on a large bed of mixed greens topped with 1 tbsp. of chopped walnuts and drizzled with red wine vinaigrette.
1 large sweet potato (8 oz.) topped with fresh ground cinnamon and 1 tbsp. of Brummel and Brown butter.
12 oz. of juice or sports drink.

tuna, chicken, or salmon salad: mix an 8-oz. can with 1 tbsp. of real mayonnaise, pepper, a splash of lemon juice, and 1 tsp. of olive oil. Serve over a bed of romaine lettuce and a variety of vegetables of your choice.
1½ cups of whole-wheat pasta with ¼ cup of Parmesan cheese.
16 oz. of 100 percent juice.

8-oz. chicken breast brushed lightly with barbecue sauce.
1 medium sweet potato (8 oz.); add ground cinnamon and 1 tbsp. of butter (try Brummel and Brown).
1 cup of corn, fresh or canned, no salt added.

2 cups of whole-wheat pasta topped with red sauce and 8 oz. of extralean ground turkey breast (try Honeysuckle).
2 cups of steamed broccoli (top with ¼ cup of Parmesan cheese).

grilled chicken fajitas: use 2 small whole-wheat tortillas (try La Tortilla Factory) and 8 oz. of chicken breast. Add ½ cup of beans (black or pinto), ¼ cup of light cheese, ¼–½ cup of salsa, and ¼ cup of diced onions and green peppers (optional).

8-oz. extralean turkey burger (try Honeysuckle extralean ground turkey) on a wheat bun.
side salad: a bed of mixed romaine and spinach leaves with light Italian dressing; add any vegetables you like.
12 oz. of 100 percent juice

8 oz. of grilled fish with 2 cups of lentils and broiled tomatoes (slice 1 whole tomato) topped with ¼ cup of fresh mozzarella cheese.
12 oz. of juice.

8 oz. of shrimp or crawfish, stir-fried with mushrooms, spinach, onions, and minced garlic in 2 tsp. of olive oil and a splash of soy sauce. Serve over 1 cup of brown rice or 1 cup of whole-wheat pasta.
2 cups of grilled or sautéed asparagus.
12 oz. of juice.

2 whole-wheat tortilla wraps (try La Tortilla Factory) with 8 oz. of turkey or chicken, (for turkey, try Honeysuckle's extralean turkey breast), 1 thin deli slice of cheese, and cooked vegetables (onions, green peppers, tomatoes).
steamed broccoli and cauliflower.
8–12 oz. of juice.

pita pocket sandwich: stuff 8 oz. of your favorite lean protein (turkey, chicken, tuna, or extralean ground beef) into 1 whole-wheat pita (2 pockets). Add fresh spinach leaves, sliced red peppers, and a drizzle of light vinaigrette dressing.
side salad topped with 1 tbsp. of almonds or walnuts and light dressing.

protein shake: mix 40 g whey protein powder (should contain no more than 4 g of carbohydrates per 20 g) with 12 oz. of skim or soy milk, 2 tbsp. of ground flaxseed, 2 tbsp. of peanut butter, and 1 cup of fresh or frozen berries (no sugar added). Add ice and blend.

Dinner Options

8 oz. of grilled tuna or salmon with portobello mushrooms and red peppers, grilled or roasted, with 2 tsp. of olive oil and seasonings. Serve over 1 cup of brown rice.

shrimp-veggie lo-mein: 8 oz. of grilled shrimp (grill in a wok or a pan with about 1 tbsp. of olive oil). Serve over 2 cups of whole-wheat pasta (long; try Barilla or Hodgson Mill) and mixed sautéed vegetables (broccoli, zucchini, squash, tomatoes, and onions). You can add these to the wok once the shrimp is cooked.

meat loaf (8 oz.); use extralean ground beef (96 percent lean).
1 large baked potato (8 oz.); add ¼ cup of low-fat shredded cheese and 2 tsp. of Brummel and Brown butter.
mixed green salad tossed with 1 tbsp. of light vinaigrette dressing.

4 shrimp and chicken kabobs, made with any vegetables you like (mushrooms, onions, and peppers work well).
1 large sweet potato (8 oz.); add cinnamon and 2 tsp. of Brummel and Brown butter.
grilled or sautéed vegetables of choice.

turkey breast fillet (8 oz.)

1 large baked potato (8 oz.); add 2 tsp. of Brummel and Brown butter and ⅓ cup of low-fat cheddar cheese.

2 cups of steamed broccoli with ¼ cup of Parmesan cheese.

pork tenderloin medallions (8 oz.).

2 cups of whole-wheat fettuccini noodles (add 2 tbsp. of minced garlic, 1 tbsp. of olive oil, and ¼ cup of Parmesan cheese).

2 cups of asparagus, steamed with a splash each of lemon juice and balsamic vinegar.

protein shake: mix 40 g whey protein powder (should contain no more than 4 g of carbohydrates per 20 g) with 12 oz. of skim or soy milk, 1–2 tbsp. of ground flaxseed, 2 tbsp. of peanut butter, and 1 cup of fresh or frozen berries (no sugar added). Add ice and blend.

Meal Plans for the 4,500-Calorie Program

The meal plans below, divided into options for breakfast, lunch, dinner, and snacks, are designed so that if you eat three meals and two snacks per day, you will be ingesting 4,500 calories.

Breakfast Options

1½ cups of cooked oatmeal with 1 tbsp. of ground flaxseed (optional), or stir in 20 g of whey protein powder.

3 low-fat and/or vegetarian sausage patties (try Healthy Choice, Morningstar Farms, or Boca varieties).

16 oz. of 100 percent juice.

1 carton of Egg Beaters, scrambled, with 2 thin slices of lean ham, rolled into 2 small whole-wheat tortillas (look for at least 3 g of fiber; we like La Tortilla Factory, with 8–9 g of fiber per tortilla).

16 oz. of skim or soy milk (or 1 container of light yogurt) or 12–16 oz. of juice.

2 breakfast burritos, using small (1-oz.) whole-wheat tortillas (try La Tortilla Factory) with 5 egg whites plus 1 yolk, 2 tbsp. of salsa (optional), ⅓ cup of low-fat cheese, and ¼ cup of diced onions and green peppers.

16 oz. of skim or soy milk (or add 1 oz. of cheese to the burritos).

1 large piece of fresh fruit (an apple or a pear, 8 oz.).

3 slices of 100 percent whole-grain bread (at least 3 g of fiber per slice).

2 whole eggs plus 5 egg whites, prepared any way you like.

1 cup of applesauce (sweetened).

20 oz. of 100 percent juice.

2–3 whole-grain waffles such as Kashi or Van's 7-grain frozen waffles, or made from a whole-wheat baking mix such as Hodgson Mill, topped with 1 tbsp. of peanut butter (preferably natural).
16 oz. of skim or soy milk.
1 container of light yogurt or 1 piece of fresh fruit.

2 cups of whole-wheat pasta (yes, it can be a great breakfast, for all you pasta lovers!) drizzled with 1 tsp. of olive oil with 6 oz. of lean protein tossed in—such as chicken or shrimp (you can also sprinkle ¼ cup of light mozzarella cheese on top).
16 oz. of 100 percent juice.

grab-and-go sandwich: 2 slices of whole-grain bread, 5 slices of turkey, and a thin slice of cheese—throw it together, fold it over, and you've got a great breakfast for the road.
1 piece of fresh fruit.
20 oz. of 100 percent juice or low-fat milk.

protein shake: mix 40 g whey protein powder (should contain no more than 4 g of carbohydrates per 20 g) with 12 oz. of skim or soy milk, 2 tbsp. of peanut butter, 1–2 tbsp. of ground flaxseed, and 1 cup of fresh or frozen berries (no sugar added). Add ice and blend.

Snack Options

Anytime you are going more than four hours between meals, you should make sure that you have a snack to boost your metabolism and stabilize insulin levels. Below are some suggestions for midmorning and midafternoon snacks.

1 large red apple with 2 tbsp. of almond butter on 2 slices of whole-grain bread.

15 whole-grain crackers (e.g., woven wheat crackers) topped with sliced mozzarella cheese (approximately 1 oz.) and 1 piece of fresh fruit.

trail mix: small box of raisins with 10–12 mixed nuts and 1 cup of dried fruit.

1 cup of low-fat cottage cheese with 2 cups of fresh berries and 1 container of light yogurt.

15 low-fat chips (e.g., Sun Chips, which are high in fiber) with 4 tbsp. of bean dip or hummus and a 4-oz. chicken breast.

2 whole-wheat tortillas (try La Tortilla Factory) topped with 2 tbsp. of low-fat shredded cheddar, melted, and 3 oz. of grilled chicken. Roll up and dip into salsa and low-fat sour cream.

2 cups of Kashi GOLEAN Crunch! cereal mixed with 1 container of light yogurt.

at a smoothie store or a gym smoothie bar: Myoplex Deluxe blended with 1 percent milk (my favorite flavor: Cappuccino Ice).

protein shake: mix 40 g of whey protein powder (should contain no more than 4 g of carbohydrate per 20 g) with 8 oz. skim or soy milk and 1 tbsp. of ground flaxseed (optional). Add ice and blend.

2 squares of dark chocolate (look for at least 70 percent cocoa) with 10–12 nuts (try almonds or walnuts for added omega-3 fatty acids) and 1 piece of fresh fruit.

Lunch Options

8 oz. of seared tuna on a large bed of mixed greens topped with 1 tbsp. of chopped walnuts and drizzled with red wine vinaigrette
1 large sweet potato (8 oz.) topped with fresh ground cinnamon and 2 tbsp. of Brummel and Brown butter.
20 oz. of juice or sports drink.

tuna, chicken, or salmon salad: mix an 8-oz. can with 1 tbsp. of real mayonnaise, pepper, a splash of lemon juice, and 1 tbsp. of olive oil. Serve over a bed of romaine lettuce and a variety of vegetables of your choice.
2 cups of whole-wheat pasta with ¼ cup of Parmesan cheese.
16–20 oz. of 100 percent juice.

8-oz. chicken breast brushed lightly with barbecue sauce.
1 large sweet potato (12 oz.); add ground cinnamon and 1 tbsp. of butter (try Brummel and Brown).
2 cups of corn, fresh or canned, no salt added.

2 cups of whole-wheat pasta topped with red sauce and 8 oz. of extralean ground turkey breast (try Honeysuckle).
1–2 cups of green peas, no salt added.
12–16 oz. of juice.

grilled chicken fajitas: use 2–3 small whole-wheat tortillas (try La Tortilla Factory) and 8 oz. of chicken breast. Add 1 cup of beans (black or pinto, ⅓–½ cup to each tortilla), ¼ cup of low-fat cheese, ¼–½ cup of salsa, and ¼ cup of diced onions and green peppers (optional).
12 oz. of juice.

two 4-oz. extralean turkey burgers (try Honeysuckle extralean ground turkey) each on a wheat bun.
1 cup of beans, peas, or corn.

8 oz. of grilled fish with 2 cups of lentils or beans (any kind) and broiled tomatoes (slice 1 whole tomato) topped with ¼ cup of fresh mozzarella cheese.
16 oz. of juice.

8 oz. of shrimp or crawfish, stir-fried with mushrooms, spinach, onions, and minced garlic in 2 tsp. of olive oil and a splash of soy sauce. Serve over 1 cup of brown rice or 1 cup of whole-wheat pasta.
1 cup of green beans mixed with 1 cup of corn.
12 oz. of juice.

2 whole-wheat tortilla wraps (try La Tortilla Factory) with 8 oz. of turkey or chicken (for turkey, try Honeysuckle's extralean turkey breast), 1 thick deli slice of cheese, and cooked vegetables (onions, green peppers, tomatoes).
steamed broccoli and cauliflower.
16–20 oz. of juice.

2 pita pocket sandwiches (2 whole pitas): stuff 4 oz. of your favorite lean protein (turkey, chicken, tuna, or extralean ground beef) into each whole-wheat pita. Add fresh spinach leaves, sliced red peppers, and a drizzle of light vinaigrette dressing.
side salad topped with 1 tbsp. of almonds or walnuts and light dressing.
12 oz. of juice.

protein shake: mix 40 g of whey protein powder (should contain no more than 4 g of carbohydrates per 20 g) with 12 oz. of skim or soy milk, 2 tbsp. of ground flaxseed, 2 tbsp. of peanut butter, and 1 cup of fresh or frozen berries (no sugar added). Add ice and blend.

Dinner Options

8 oz. of grilled tuna or salmon with portobello mushrooms and red peppers, grilled or roasted, with 2 tsp. of olive oil and seasonings. Serve over 1 cup of brown rice.

shrimp-veggie lo-mein: 8 oz. of grilled shrimp (grill in a wok or a pan with about 1 tbsp. of olive oil). Serve over 2 cups of whole-wheat pasta (long; try Barilla or Hodgson Mill) and 1–1½ cups of mixed starchy vegetables (corn, peas, carrots).

meat loaf (8 oz.); use extralean ground beef (96 percent lean)
1 large baked potato (12 oz.); add ¼ cup of low-fat shredded cheese and 1 tbsp. of Brummel and Brown butter.
mixed green salad tossed with 1 tbsp. of light vinaigrette dressing.
12–16 oz. of juice.

5–6 shrimp and chicken kabobs, made with any vegetables you like (mushrooms, onions, and peppers work well).
1 large sweet potato (8 oz.); add cinnamon and 2 tsp. of Brummel and Brown butter.
grilled or sautéed vegetables of choice.
12–16 oz. of juice.

turkey breast fillet (8 oz.)

1 large baked potato (12 oz.); add 2 tsp. of Brummel and Brown butter and ⅓ cup of low-fat cheddar cheese.

steamed mixed vegetables (try corn, peas, and carrots for extra calories).

12–16 oz. of juice.

pork tenderloin medallions (8 oz.)

2 cups of whole-wheat fettuccini noodles (add 2 tbsp. of minced garlic, 1 tbsp. of olive oil, and ¼ cup of Parmesan cheese).

2 whole-wheat rolls or slices of whole-wheat bread with 1 tsp. of Brummel and Brown butter on each.

12–16 oz. of juice.

protein shake: mix 40 g of whey protein powder (should contain no more than 4 g of carbohydrates per 20 g) with 12 oz. of skim or soy milk, 1–2 tbsp. of ground flaxseed, 2 tbsp. of peanut butter, and 1 cup of fresh or frozen berries (no sugar added). Add ice and blend.

Meal Plans for the 5,000-Calorie Program

The meal plans below, divided into options for breakfast, lunch, dinner, and snacks, are designed so that if you eat three meals and two snacks per day, you will be ingesting 5,000 calories.

Breakfast Options

1½ cups of cooked oatmeal with 1 tbsp. of ground flaxseed (optional), or stir in 30 g of whey protein powder.

3 low-fat and/or vegetarian sausage patties (try Healthy Choice, Morningstar Farms, or Boca varieties).

24 oz. of 100 percent juice.

1 carton of Egg Beaters, scrambled, with 3–4 thin slices of lean ham, rolled into 2 small whole-wheat tortillas (look for at least 3 g of fiber; we like La Tortilla Factory, with 8–9 g of fiber per tortilla).

16 oz. of skim or soy milk (or 1 container of light yogurt) or 16–20 oz. of juice.

2 breakfast burritos, using small (1-oz.) whole-wheat tortillas (try La Tortilla Factory) with 5 egg whites plus 1 yolk, 2 tbsp. of salsa (optional), ¼ cup of low-fat cheese, and ¼ cup of diced onions and green peppers.

smoothie: blend 16 oz. of skim or soy milk, 1 tbsp. of peanut butter, and a small banana.

3 slices of 100 percent whole-grain bread (at least 3 g of fiber per slice).

2 whole eggs plus 5 egg whites, prepared any way you like.

2 cups of applesauce (sweetened).

20 oz. of 100 percent juice.

3 whole-grain waffles such as Kashi or Van's 7-grain frozen waffles, or made from a whole-wheat baking mix such as Hodgson Mill, topped with 1 tbsp. peanut butter (preferably natural).
20 oz. of skim milk or soy milk or 100 percent juice.
1 container of light yogurt or 1 piece of fresh fruit.

2 cups of whole-wheat pasta (yes, it can be a great breakfast, for all you pasta lovers!) drizzled with 1 tsp. of olive oil with 6 oz. of lean protein tossed in—such as chicken or shrimp (you can also sprinkle ¼ cup of light mozzarella cheese on top).
20–24 oz. of 100 percent juice.

grab-and-go sandwich: 2 slices of whole-grain bread, 5 slices of turkey, and a thin slice of cheese—throw it together, fold it over, and you've got a great breakfast for the road.
handful of nuts of choice.
20 oz. of 100 percent juice or low-fat milk.

protein shake: mix 40 g of whey protein powder (should contain no more than 4 g of carbohydrates per 20 g) with 12 oz. of skim or soy milk, 2 tbsp. of peanut butter, 1–2 tbsp. of ground flaxseed, and 1 cup of fresh or frozen berries (no sugar added). Add ice and blend.

Snack Options

Anytime you are going more than four hours between meals, you should make sure that you have a snack to boost your metabolism and stabilize insulin levels. Below are some suggestions for midmorning and midafternoon snacks.

2 pieces of fresh fruit with 2 tbsp. of almond butter on 2 slices of whole-grain bread.

15 whole-grain crackers (e.g., woven wheat crackers) topped with sliced mozzarella (approximately 1 oz.) and 2–3 slices of lean deli meat (turkey, ham, or roast beef) or 3 oz. of canned tuna packed in water.

trail mix: small box of raisins with 10–12 mixed nuts and 1–2 cups of dried fruit.

1 cup of low-fat cottage cheese with 2 cups of fresh berries, 1 container of light yogurt, and 1 tbsp. of peanut butter.

15 low-fat chips (e.g., Sun Chips, which are high in fiber) with 4 tbsp. of bean dip or hummus and a 4-oz. chicken breast.

2 whole-wheat tortillas (try La Tortilla Factory) topped with 2 tbsp. of low-fat shredded cheddar, melted, and 5 oz. of grilled chicken. Roll up and dip into salsa and low-fat sour cream.

2 cups of Kashi GOLEAN Crunch! cereal mixed with 2 containers of light yogurt.

at a smoothie store or a gym smoothie bar: Myoplex Deluxe blended with 1 percent milk (my favorite flavor: Cappuccino Ice)

protein shake: mix 40 g of whey protein powder (should contain no more than 4 g of carbohydrate per 20 g) with 8 oz. of skim or soy milk and 1 tbsp. of ground flaxseed (optional). Add ice and blend.

2 squares of dark chocolate (look for at least 70 percent cocoa) with 10–12 nuts (try almonds or walnuts for added omega-3 fatty acids) and 1 piece of fresh fruit.

Lunch Options

8–10 oz. of seared tuna on a large bed of mixed greens topped with 1 tbsp. of chopped walnuts and drizzled with red wine vinaigrette.
1 large sweet potato (8 oz.) topped with fresh ground cinnamon and 2 tbsp. of Brummel and Brown butter.
20 oz. of juice or sports drink.

tuna, chicken, or salmon salad: mix 1½ 5-oz. cans of tuna with 1 tbsp. of real mayonnaise, pepper, a splash of lemon juice, and 1 tbsp. of olive oil. Serve over a bed of romaine lettuce and a variety of vegetables of your choice.
2 cups of whole-wheat pasta with ¼ cup of Parmesan cheese.
16–20 oz. of 100 percent juice.

8-oz. chicken breast brushed lightly with barbecue sauce.
1 large sweet potato (12 oz.); add ground cinnamon and 1 tbsp. of butter (try Brummel and Brown).
2 cups of corn, fresh or canned, no salt added.

2 cups of whole-wheat pasta topped with red sauce and 8 oz. of extralean ground turkey breast (try Honeysuckle).
1–2 cups of green peas, no salt added.
12–16 oz. of juice.

grilled chicken fajitas: use 3 small whole-wheat tortillas (try La Tortilla Factory) and 8 oz. of chicken breast. Add 1 cup of beans (black or pinto, ⅓–½ cup to each tortilla, ¼ cup of low-fat cheese, ¼–½ cup of salsa, and ¼ cup of diced onions and green peppers (optional).
12 oz. of juice.

two 4-oz. extralean turkey burgers (try Honeysuckle extralean ground turkey) each on a wheat bun.
1 cup of beans, peas, or corn.
12 oz. of juice.

8 oz. of grilled fish with 2 cups of lentils or beans (any kind) and broiled tomatoes (slice 1 whole tomato) topped with ¼ cup of fresh mozzarella cheese.
16–20 oz. of juice.

8 oz. of shrimp or crawfish, stir-fried with mushrooms, spinach, onions, and minced garlic in 2 tsp. olive oil and a splash of soy sauce. Serve over 1 cup of brown rice.
1 cup of green beans mixed with 1 cup of corn.
16–20 oz. of juice.

2 whole-wheat tortilla wraps (try La Tortilla Factory) with 8 oz. of turkey or chicken (for turkey, try Honeysuckle's extralean turkey breast), 1 thick deli slice of cheese, and cooked vegetables (onions, green peppers, tomatoes).
steamed broccoli and cauliflower.
20–24 oz. of juice.

2 pita pocket sandwiches (2 whole pitas): stuff 4 oz. of your favorite lean protein (turkey, chicken, tuna, or extralean ground beef) into each whole-wheat pita. Add fresh spinach leaves, sliced red peppers, and a drizzle of light vinaigrette dressing.
side salad topped with 1 tbsp. of almonds or walnuts and light dressing.
12 oz. of juice.

protein shake: mix 40 g of whey protein powder (should contain no more than 4 g of carbohydrates per 20 g) with 12 oz. of skim or soy milk, 2 tbsp. of ground flaxseed, 2 tbsp. of peanut butter, and 1 cup of fresh or frozen berries (no sugar added). Add ice and blend.

Dinner Options

8 oz. of grilled tuna or salmon with portobello mushrooms and red peppers, grilled or roasted, with 2 tsp. of olive oil and seasonings. Serve over 1 cup of brown rice.
12–16 oz. of juice.

shrimp-veggie lo-mein: 8 oz. of grilled shrimp (grill in a wok or a pan with about 1 tbsp. of olive oil). Serve over 2 cups of whole-wheat pasta (long; try Barilla or Hodgson Mill) and 1–1½ cups of mixed starchy vegetables (corn, peas, carrots)
12–16 oz. of juice.

meat loaf (8 oz.); use extralean ground beef (96 percent lean).
1 large baked potato (12 oz.); add ¼ cup of low-fat shredded cheese and 1 tbsp. of Brummel and Brown butter if you like.
mixed green salad tossed with 1 tbsp. of light vinaigrette dressing.
12–16 oz. of juice.

5–6 shrimp and chicken kabobs, made with any vegetables you like (mushrooms, onions, and peppers work well).

1 large sweet potato (8 oz); add cinnamon and 2 tsp. of Brummel and Brown butter.

grilled or sautéed vegetables of choice.

12–16 oz. of juice.

turkey breast fillet (8 oz.)

1 large baked potato (12 oz.); add 2 tsp. of Brummel and Brown butter and ⅓ cup of low-fat cheddar cheese.

steamed mixed vegetables (try corn, peas, and carrots for extra calories).

12–16 oz. of juice.

pork tenderloin medallions (8 oz.)

2 cups of whole-wheat fettuccini noodles (add 2 tbsp. of minced garlic, 1 tbsp. of olive oil, and ¼ cup of Parmesan cheese).

2 whole-wheat rolls or slices of whole-wheat bread with 1 tsp. of Brummel and Brown butter on each.

1 cup of steamed vegetables of your choice.

12–16 oz. of juice.

protein shake: mix 40 g of whey protein powder (should contain no more than 4 g of carbohydrates per 20 g) with 12 oz. of skim or soy milk, 1–2 tbsp. of ground flaxseed, 2 tbsp. of peanut butter, and 1 cup of fresh or frozen berries (no sugar added). Add ice and blend.

6

Lean and Hard Performance Supplementation

Maximize Your Workout to Build Lean Muscle

I once heard a well-known nutritionist say, "If two out of three people in America are on a diet, then why are 67 percent of us still overweight or obese?" This is how I would rephrase this statement for people who are trying to get fit: If our gyms and health food stores are filled with hundreds of products designed to increase muscle and workout efficiency—and millions of people are using them—then why is it so difficult to get lean and hard? Why aren't people getting the results that these products promise?

To use the language of the computer age, the problem is not the "hardware," or the products. The problem is the "software," a system that shows you how to use these products *synergistically* before, during, and after your workout for maximum energy, repair, and muscle building.

The Need for a Balanced Program

I know how frustrated and confused people are about substances such as creatine monohydrate, maltodextrin, and whey protein powder. I have worked with countless individuals who take these supplements but can't get them to deliver the promised results in stamina, power, and muscle gain. When I was interviewed in *Muscle and Fitness* magazine about how I had used performance nutrition supplementation to put additional lean muscle on Michael Spinks, I got 750 letters in response. They all said pretty much the same thing: "I've been taking muscle- and power-building products for years and I've tried everything on the market, but nothing seems to work for me. What am I doing wrong?"

Even professional boxers, football players, and other athletes whose million-dollar-a-year careers depend upon their developing and maintaining a significant amount of lean muscle don't always get the results they want.

The secret is the system—how all these performance nutrition supplements can combine to create a foolproof muscle-building program in conjunction with the high-intensity workout and high-performance food program.

In any sport that requires strength and power—such as boxing, bodybuilding, football, or baseball— you will find athletes who have tried all kinds of pro hormones, such as steroids and testosterone, and supplements (both legal and illegal) during the off-season, trying to create a leaner, more muscular body. In fact, over the last few years the media have reported some pretty alarming stories about steroid use and the athletes who have compromised their health— and sometimes even ruined their careers—using them. Using even legal pro hormones, especially if they haven't been around long enough for people to see the long-term impact on health, can be risky. In 1998, I worked with a talented twenty-two-year-old player preparing for his tryout for the Canadian Football League. I discovered that he was taking a supplement called Androstendione, a muscle-building pro hormone that performs in the body very much like testosterone. This drug has since been taken off the market because of its side effects, but it was legal at the time and could be bought in many health food stores.

To support his training regimen, he was taking 100 milligrams of this pro hormone two times a day, double the recommended dose. Like a lot of people I've worked with, he assumed that if 50 milligrams was good, then he could get double the results in half the time with 100 milligrams

Everyone has to have a health screening before he or she can come into my program. I'd just read a research paper about the potential downside of Androstendione, so I was waiting to see what the doctor would find. When he tested this young rookie, he discovered that his LDL, bad cholesterol, was 200 (doctors begin treating you for high cholesterol if your LDL is over 130). His HDL, good cholesterol, was only 26, almost half what it should have been for a healthy person his age. These results matched with what the study said about the drug causing a "reverse cholesterol" pattern.

Things looked even worse when he did a cardiopulmonary stress test. Since I'd just turned forty-eight, I'd taken this test the day before. When I was finished, it took only thirty seconds for my heart rate to come back to baseline—one of the best recovery rates the physiologist had ever seen. With the double dose of pro hormone the rookie had been taking, it took him over half an hour to come back to baseline. And he was less than half my age.

We took him off the supplement immediately because his cardiovascular system was taking a beating, which would have made him vulnerable for heart disease later in life. Not only that, we knew that the elevated testosterone levels this drug was causing would make him test positive for steroids when he tried out for the team. All of his talent and hard work and the years of practice he'd put into the sport would have been wasted and he would have been finished before he even got his shot at the pros.

Why Not Use the Latest Wonder Drug?

Every year brings some new muscle-building wonder drug to the market, and many people start using it. When the product fails to prove safe over the long run, they find their health endangered. When used without medical supervision, many steroidlike pro hormones have been known to cause liver and kidney damage, high cholesterol, low HDL, premature balding, aggressive behavior in both genders, and cystic acne.

Even if the product has been shown to be "safe" in certain studies, taking supplements such as Androstendione, DHEA, and secretagogues without the proper program of training, timing, and nutrition is simply a waste of money and a danger to your health.

I prefer to stay with what has been successful in my own work with athletes over the last decade. The supplements I describe in this chapter—creatine monohydrate, maltodextrin, whey protein, and L-glutamine—have been around for a while. But, until now, a cohesive system for using them to build muscle rapidly and safely has not been available. When I asked James Tebbe, M.D., the Ochsner Health System family medicine physician and medical director of the Elmwood Fitness Center, who evaluates individuals who wish to take my program, to give me his take on the safety of the supplements described in this book, he wrote the following:

"Surveys show that more than half of the U.S. adult population uses vitamins and dietary supplements, to the tune of $18 billion in 2003 (nearly triple the $6.5 billion spent in 1996). Unfortunately, false claims (such as "cure-all" and "totally safe") and clever advertising ("all natural" and "money-back guarantee") entice buyers into purchasing items with little evidence of health benefits. However, there is an *abundance* of scientific evidence in the medical literature supporting the safety and efficacy of the four supplements recommended by Mackie in this program.

"Remember: balance is the key! More is not always better. Anything can become dangerous if you take too much of it. When the supplements that Mackie recommends in this program are used as he suggests, and under medical supervision, *you will get results*."

In conjunction with the high-intensity exercises and high-performance food program described in this book, this performance nutrition supplementation schedule will enable you to maximize your workout and pack on the muscle. This system is based not only on the results of my twenty-five-year career working with thousands of top athletes but is also one of the only university-tested, high-performance exercise/nutrition/supplementation programs of which I am aware.

No matter who you are or what kind of shape you are in, the performance nutrition supplementation described in this chapter will deliver on its promise to build a significant amount of lean muscle in only 24 workouts spread over 6 weeks.

Learn Why Nutrition Alone Is Not Enough

A lot of people say to me, "Mackie, why do you want me to take supplements? Isn't just eating a lot of good food and some extra protein enough to fuel my workout?"

If you are performing high-intensity exercise to build muscle, food alone—no matter how good your nutritional program—will not be able to give you everything you need. If you didn't take performance nutrition supplements, the calories required to increase, maintain, and repair muscle would be so enormous that you would have to eat between 5,500 and 6,500 calories per day!

If we look at the scientific theory, to build even one pound of muscle a week, you would need to ingest roughly an extra 19 grams of protein per day, beyond your normal protein requirements. And you would have to eat three to four times that many carbohydrates because carbs provide energy for the workout, helping the body to store available protein instead of burning it as fuel.

It's unrealistic to expect that you'd be able to efficiently turn all that food into muscle. Beyond a certain point, the body just can't efficiently digest such a large quantity of meat, grains, vegetables, fruit, and so on, because all of these things take time and energy to be broken down and delivered where they are needed in the body. So, a lot of those calories would be either excreted or turned into stored fat, which is the *opposite* of what you want. Meanwhile, your digestive system would be in a constant state of overwork and stress. You would likely feel bloated and nauseous during your workout.

When you are involved in a high-performance workout, you need a performance nutrition regimen that can get the fuel you require into your cells and muscle tissue *as quickly and efficiently as possible*.

That's the beauty of performance nutrition supplements. They are designed to be very easy to absorb, causing little digestive stress in the body. When you add performance nutrition supplements to your food plan, you may only require between 2,500 and 3,000 calories per day (total) to keep your body's energy system running at peak capacity.

When you take these supplements, you will be able to train longer and harder and at a higher level of performance. You will also reduce your risk of injury and recover from your workout at a faster rate.

Performance nutrition supplementation should never *replace* the three meals and three snacks I am asking you to eat throughout the day, but should be taken in addition to them, according to the schedule I give you in this chapter.

Check with Your Doctor before You Begin

Before I describe to you the types of supplements you will be taking during your Lean and Hard Program, I strongly recommend that you work in conjunction with your doctor. This is especially important if you have any preexisting condition or potential for any disease.

Working without your physician's approval and guidance would be like trying to drive your car in the dark without headlights—a recipe for disaster. When I asked Dr. Tebbe to comment on the importance of this, he wrote the following:

"I cannot overemphasize the importance of consulting with your personal physician before starting an exercise program. This is especially true, not just for those with known medical conditions (such as diabetes, high blood pressure, or heart disease), but also for the deconditioned (or 'out of shape') person. We would never plan a major renovation on a home, or a complete overhaul of a car engine, without seeking advice from a professional. We should give our bodies (and our health) the same consideration. The purpose of this type of consultation is not to disqualify someone from participating in a certain exercise program. On the contrary: I'm *delighted* when patients take our advice, and begin to integrate proper nutrition and exercise into the treatment and prevention of disease.

"Our relationship with Mackie and his fitness team is a very collaborative one, with the mutual objective of improving the general health and well-being of the client. Our job is to ensure that we set *realistic* goals that can be achieved *safely*."

Let me caution you that this type of performance supplementation protocol should only be followed if you are engaged in a program of high-intensity exercise. While it is always important to one's health to take supplemental nutrients such as vitamins and antioxidants, loading up daily on substances such as creatine monohydrate, maltodextrin, whey protein powder, and L-glutamine without a strategic plan and medical approval does not make sense. This supplementation protocol is designed with a specific purpose in mind: to support the Lean and Hard Workout Program.

Performance Nutrition Supplements: The Supersynergistic Four

To help get the absolute maximum muscle-building capacity from each of your workouts, I am asking you to take four types of performance nutrition supplements. Since they are designed to work in combination with one another, I call them my Supersynergistic Four.

1. Creatine monohydrate to increase energy availability and retard the breakdown of muscle tissue during the workout.

2. A whey protein drink containing sufficient essential (not manufactured by the body) and nonessential (made by the body) amino acids. Whey, a "fast" (easily digestible) protein, provides a quick influx of amino acids, the building blocks of protein, to help preserve muscle fibers during a workout and to replace proteins in muscle fibers following a workout, facilitating muscle repair and growth.

3. L-glutamine, an amino acid that is essential to accelerating recovery between workouts, increasing lean muscle mass, and improving immune function.

4. Maltodextrin, a fast-absorbing carbohydrate powder taken both before and after the workout to provide energy, minimize loss of muscle mass, and aid in recovery.

Another advantage to these products is that they are reasonably priced, although I suggest not purchasing the cheapest generic brands. In my experience using these types of performance nutrition supplements, you get what you pay for. The better brands generally have superior-grade ingredients and more accurate labeling. For that reason, I recommend that you stick with the major sports and fitness supplement companies such as Unipro, Cell-Tech, Pro Lab, Muscletech, or EAS. These products can be purchased in your local health food store, GNC-type store, or gym. These supplements come in a powder form and should be dissolved in water or juice and taken sixty to thirty minutes before your workout. During a meal or following a workout, dissolve them in water, juice, low-fat milk, or soy milk.

The Importance of Protein and Amino Acids to Support High-Intensity Training

Protein is one of the most important nutrients needed to support a high-intensity workout. As we saw in chapter 3, protein is the king of nutrients.

- It makes up the structural basis for all body tissues and is involved in their development, growth, and repair.
- It is a crucial component in the regulation of metabolism. Enzymes control all metabolic reactions and all enzymes are formed from protein.
- It is a vital source of energy. Protein is so important that no other nutrient can take its place. During periods of starvation or scarcity, the body will cannibalize its own protein stores (muscle tissue) for energy.
- It is essential for the production of hormones such as insulin, human growth hormone, and glucagon.
- Protein breaks down into amino acids and amino acids break down into nitrogen. When your body has a nitrogen deficit, you will lose muscle mass. When you have a positive nitrogen balance, you gain muscle mass.
- The branch chain amino acids (BCAA) found in the whey protein powder I recommend "results in greater net muscle protein synthesis," according to a recent study done at the University of Texas.

The body is in a constant dynamic flux, synthesizing nutrients from protein and excreting them as waste materials once they have been used as an energy source. Unlike fat, which it can store in large amounts, the body stores very little excess protein. Therefore, if you are following a high-intensity training (HIT) regimen, it is crucial to make sure that your nutrition program includes adequate amounts of protein and supplements containing the amino acids found in proteins. Only in this way can you ensure the following.

- An increase in your energy availability during high-intensity training
- A decrease in the amount of muscle tissue broken down during your workout
- The efficient repair of muscle following your workout

A Note to Women

When I state that this program is going to build muscularity, this does not mean that you will end up with an unfeminine body, bulging with muscles. Because of the types of hormones involved in building a large, muscled body, female bodybuilders have to go to great extremes to create their large physiques. While male readers will bulk up on the Lean and Hard Program, women will achieve a leaner, firmer physique with less body fat and more well-defined curves. The women who were part of the original Lean and Hard Study done at Louisiana State University Health Care Network looked svelte and lean following their six weeks on the program.

When consulting your doctor about the program, ask about the proper amount of calcium needed when consuming supplemental protein or creatine monohydrate. The normal range for calcium intake is between 1,000 and 1,500 milligrams per day (dietary and/or supplement). This requirement may increase based on your physician's determination. Ingesting larger amounts of protein can increase your phosphorous level, which may leach calcium from the body. If you increase your calcium intake, you will also need your doctor to adjust your magnesium and vitamin D levels accordingly. (These two substances are often included in your calcium supplement.)

Creatine: Your Energy Engine for High-Intensity Training and Muscle Repair

Because of its ability to help increase and sustain muscle energy levels during HIT, creatine monohydrate is one of the most widely used supplements for strength and power athletes. It also helps accelerate the recovery process between workouts.

Despite its popularity, I have found that creatine is also one of the most misused supplements on the market. In my experience, 90 percent of the people who buy it don't understand what it does or how to effectively use it. When I gave a lecture to a university track team, I found that many of them were taking creatine monohydrate, yet not one could tell me how much creatine he should be using or how to use it to improve his running performance. They were just swigging it haphazardly when they happened to think about it during the day.

Here's an example of why we don't want you to take more than the prescribed amount of creatine in the supplemental plan. I remember one extremely gifted young middle linebacker who was part of our NFL draft preparation program. He was 6' 6" tall and 290 pounds of muscle. We discovered that he was taking 20 grams of creatine monohydrate a day. Normally, the loading dose is 20 grams per day for three to five days during the training cycle. After that, you drop down to three to five grams per day because 5 grams is the maximum your body can absorb once it has become saturated. Anything you take over and above that amount will be excreted by the kidneys.

Since this young man had decided that more was better, he had continued with his 20 grams of creatine monohydrate a day for over a year. When my doctors tested his kidney function, his creatinine level, one of the markers for kidney function, came up abnormal due to the excessive amount of creatine he was ingesting every day. We asked him to stop taking it for one day to allow his system to clear. When we retested him twenty-four hours later, his creatine level had returned to normal. If we hadn't caught this, the NFL doctors might have assumed there was something potentially wrong with his kidney function and would have investigated further.

Creatine and Your Health

When using creatine, make sure that you are in good health. It is always a good idea to check with your doctor first if in doubt about whether or not you should use this or any other supplement.

The safety and effectiveness of creatine monohydrate is well established because numerous studies have explored its effects on people involved in high-performance training and sports.

Medicine and Science in Sports and Exercise reported on a study of healthy people who had been taking creatine from ten months to five years. It found no difference in kidney function when they were compared to healthy people not taking creatine.

Similar results were obtained in a study published in the *International Journal of Sports Nutrition and Exercise Metabolism*. Researchers followed twenty-three healthy members of an NCAA Division II American college football team (aged nineteen to twenty-four) who were taking 5 to 20 grams of creatine monohydrate daily and studied the effects from 3 months to 5.6 years. When compared to a control group not taking creatine, these college students showed "no long-term harmful effects on kidney or liver function."

Some athletes are concerned about whether creatine monohydrate causes cramping. One of the doctors who reviewed this book said that a few of his clients had experienced some cramping while taking creatine. A recent study in the *Journal of Strength and Conditioning Research*, which involved high-performance swimmers, reported mild "gastrointestinal discomfort in swimmers who ingested creatine with large quantities of glucose polymers." In my own experience, if an athlete stays properly hydrated during his or her workout, cramping should not occur. However, some people are more sensitive to the glucose polymer/creatine combination than others. If you do find yourself cramping, either decrease your daily dose of creatine monohydrate from 5 milligrams to 3 milligrams or stop using it until you consult with your physician.

Taking creatine before a workout may actually cause a decrease in exercise-related problems. According to a study performed by Dr. Richard B. Kreider, the leading international expert on creatine: "In fact, there is recent evidence that creatine may lessen heat stress and reduce the susceptibility to musculoskeletal injuries among athletes engaged in training."

A recent article published by the National Strength and Conditioning Association stated: "Because creatine is only effective in short duration, high-intensity, and repeated-bout maximal exercises, the fatigue-delaying properties of the supplement may allow athletes to train more intensely, which can ultimately lead to greater increases in muscle mass, strength, and power, but not in flexibility or endurance."

Another interesting study by the School of Human Kinetics at Laurentian University reported the effectiveness of creatine on rebuilding muscle mass in older men, aged fifty-nine to seventy-six. As we age, we often lose muscle mass, a process called sarcopenia. When men in this age group followed a program of resistance training supplemented with creatine monohydrate, their deficits in muscle mass when compared to younger men were eliminated.

Since the Lean and Hard Workout is not based on endurance (cardiovascular) activities but on brief intervals of high-intensity exercise, creatine monohydrate is the ideal supplement to supply your energy needs.

Research has also been conducted to discover if creatine monohydrate has similar effects on both men and women. A 2004 study published by *Medicine and Science in Sports and Exercise* showed that proportionately equal amounts of creatine taken by male and female athletes during comparable bouts of high-intensity resistance exercise created an increase in lean muscle and greater energy in both genders. Because of their hormonal makeup, however, men had more of a tendency to bulk up, while women became stronger and leaner.

What Creatine Can Do for You

The benefits of creatine include the following:

- It increases strength, enabling you to get more out of your workout.
- It builds lean body mass, which allows greater force to be used during weight training.
- It increases the volume of muscle cells, resulting in their ability to store more nutrients and water.
- It facilitates faster recovery following your workout, allowing for more frequent training sessions and more intensity.

How Creatine Works in the Body

Creatine naturally occurs in animal protein such as fish, poultry, beef, and pork. For example, there are 2 grams of creatine per pound in salmon, 3 to 4.5 grams per pound in herring, 2 grams per pound in beef, and 2.3 grams per pound in pork. Creatine is created in the liver by a chemical process that combines several amino acids. Since the body can synthesize about 2 grams of creatine per day, under normal circumstance we normally stay in creatine balance. However, when we are involved in activities such as high-intensity training, we may benefit from up to 5 grams per day.

When creatine is absorbed into muscle cells, some of it binds to water molecules, which results in "cell volumization" (enlargement). When billions of individual muscle cells become larger, the entire muscle increases in size and strength.

The remaining creatine monohydrate binds to phosphate molecules, resulting in something known as "phosphocreatine," which eventually produces the chemical ATP that provides the energy for muscle contraction. The more phosphocreatine stored in your muscle, the more potential you have to produce ATP, the kind of energy you need to support your high-intensity workout.

My program suggests that you take 5 grams of creatine monohydrate four times a day for three days in order to saturate your muscle tissue with sufficient energy for your high-intensity training. Once your muscles are saturated, you will need to take 3 to 5 grams of creatine only once a day to sustain the maximum benefits (see the supplement schedule in chapter 7).

These doses are based on research by Dr. Richard B. Kreider at the Sport Nutrition Laboratory at Baylor University. He reports the results in "Sports Applications of Creatine," published by the university's Center for Exercise, Nutrition, and Preventive Health Research. Dr. Kreider recommends that "athletes take creatine with a high carbohydrate drink (e.g., juice or a concentrated carbohydrate solution) or with a carbohydrate/protein supplement in order to increase insulin and promote creatine uptake."

The Best Form of Creatine to Take

When taking creatine to improve athletic performance, it's important to use a product that is categorized as pharmaceutical grade. The majority of studies conducted on creatine have evaluated pharmacological-grade creatine monohydrate in oral or intravenous phosphocreatine formulations or in powder form. Since creatine is a very popular supplement, a variety of different forms have been marketed, such as creatine citrate, creatine bars, creatine candy, liquid creatine, creatine gum, and effervescent creatine. Many of these forms of creatine claim to be better than creatine monohydrate. However, there is no research data that indicate that any of these forms of creatine increase creatine uptake to the muscle better than creatine monohydrate. For example, a recent study by Dr. Richard Krieder indicated that liquid creatine did not improve muscle creatine stores.

There are three primary sources for creatine: Germany, the United States, and China. Independent testing has revealed that Chinese sources of creatine may have less purity and/or contain higher amounts of contaminants such as dihydrotriazine and/or creatinine. The best raw source of creatine monohydrate appears to be from Germany, a product known as Degussa's Creapure. In general, however, make sure that you purchase pharmaceutical-grade creatine monohydrate that is free from contaminants and has been produced in facilities that are inspected and that adhere to the FDA's good manufacturing practice guidelines.

Do Women Respond Differently to Creatine than Men?

Some of the initial studies of creatine suggested that women did not respond as well to creatine supplementation as men. However, recent studies, including those conducted by Dr. Kreider, have shown that women do experience muscle gains from creatine supplementation. Kreider reports, "In our research, we have found that women typically observe ergogenic benefit following short-term supplementation [with creatine]. However, gains in body mass and fat-free mass are generally not as rapid as men. Nevertheless, women do gain strength and muscle mass over time during training."

Our original Lean and Hard Study showed that the women in our program who followed our HIT workout, nutritional program, and performance nutrition supplementation protocol (creatine, maltodextrin, whey protein, vitamins/minerals, and antioxidants) did experience significant muscle gains, becoming much leaner, losing inches, and dropping fat.

Whey Protein: An Important Training Tool

Whey protein is the number one protein choice to minimize muscle breakdown during exercise and speed recovery from a high-intensity training regimen for many reasons.

- Whey protein has a full spectrum of essential and nonessential amino acids, including the branch chain amino acids (BCCA) leucine, iso-leucine, and valine, which are critical to prevention of muscle loss during intense training.
- When ingested after a workout, whey increases and stabilizes anabolic hormones, increases gains in lean muscle, and speeds fat loss.
- Whey is derived from calcium-rich milk products. Foods with a high calcium content support bone strength and increase the burning of fat.
- Whey helps the muscles to recover more quickly from the stress of exercise.
- Whey gives strong support to the immune system. Whey proteins contain high levels of the amino acid cysteine, which is needed to help the body produce glutathione, a powerful antioxidant that plays a key role in maintaining immune health. In fact, one of the first symptoms often noticed in individuals with autoimmune diseases, such as HIV, is a decline in glutathione levels.
- Due to its high amino acid and glutamine content, whey supports gastro-

intestinal health and offers relief from digestive distress such as cramps, bloating, and diarrhea.

- Two major proteins in whey, lactoferrin and lactoferricin, function as antioxidants.

How Whey Protein Maximizes High-Intensity Training

Most people believe that exercise builds muscle. This is not true—exercise merely stresses muscle tissue enough to break it down somewhat. Muscle "growth" occurs during the repair and recovery time following exercise. Therefore, the nutrients you ingest before, during, and after exercise—especially the type and amount of protein—become vitally important in the creation of stronger and larger muscles.

Here is how it works: during your HIT session, you might experience breakdown of muscle tissue, but you do not want to use it as an energy source. For this reason, ingesting the whey/maltodextrin mixture before your workout within a sixty- to thirty-minute window becomes crucial. That gives your body enough protein "fuel" to protect the muscle mass you already have.

Following your HIT session, damaged tissue will be recycled into new muscle fibers, a process known as "protein turnover." Since this repair process is never 100 percent efficient, you need a quick influx of amino acids to help replace damaged proteins.

In both of these scenarios, the *digestibility* of your protein source is your most important consideration. While fish, poultry, beef, and pork are all excellent sources of protein, animal proteins take a fairly long time to digest and are slow to release in the body. For this reason, you need a more quickly available protein source to help efficiently support your workout and the repair and rebuilding of muscle tissue following it.

Whey protein, which has a full spectrum of both essential and nonessential amino acids, is your best choice to provide the raw materials to support your workout and recovery. I ask you to take whey instead of casein, soy, or other types of protein powders because whey is known as a "fast" protein source, which means that it is easily digestible. Therefore, it can get amino acids, building blocks of muscle tissue, into your muscles quickly to make them readily available during and after your workout. A study published in the *International Journal of Sport Nutrition and Exercise Metabolism* also supports the digestive efficiency of whey protein when taken before a workout: "The rapid absorption of WP in the first 3 to 5 h accounted for the vast majority of amino acid absorption in the order of 8 to 10 g/h (grams/hour)." The easy digestibility of whey has been proven in research by the National Academy of Sciences, which tested it against other protein sources, such as casein.

Whey also promotes anabolism, a metabolic environment that increases your body's ability to build more muscle. An article titled "Protein Ingestion prior to

Strength Exercise Affects Blood Hormones and Metabolism," published in *Medicine and Science in Sports and Exercise*, showed that the consumption of whey protein prior to bouts of strength training enhanced the levels of the anabolic hormones HGH and testosterone, as well as creating levels of insulin favorable to efficient protein metabolism. Another article, titled "Influence of Nutrition on Response to Resistance Training," published by *Medicine and Science in Sports and Exercise*, states: "Amino acid availability is critical to the control of muscle protein metabolism. Thus, a meal or a supplement containing protein or amino acids will influence muscle protein." This article also compares the efficiency of whey protein and casein in repairing muscle and increasing strength following HIT. Of the two, it was concluded that whey protein is the most quickly assimilated and most readily available protein to ingest following a workout.

"Ingestion of Casein and Whey Proteins Result in Muscle Anabolism after Resistance Exercise," also published in *Medicine and Science in Sports and Exercise*, compared the results of giving subjects involved in HIT exercise either casein or whey 60 to 30 minutes before exercise and not more than 120 minutes after exercise. This study showed two things: (1) following resistance exercise, whey "stimulates net muscle protein accretion by supplying the essential amino acids necessary for muscle anabolism" (muscle building) and (2) whey protein was more easily digested than casein, making it a "fast," or readily available, protein for HIT exercise. An article published in *Medicine and Science in Sports and Exercise* also backs up the importance of taking whey before a workout: "Consuming 25 grams of whey and caseinate proteins 30 minutes before a heavy STS [strength training session] will provide the muscles a more anabolic environment by increasing the serum I levels during STS and possibly by increased T (testosterone) uptake into the muscle, but this needs further research."

A wide range of excellent whey powders is available in health food stores. The best type to buy is labeled "cross microfiltration whey isolate." This process filters out fat, lactose, and cholesterol. IsoPure Whey Isolate is one example of this type of whey protein powder. Always read the label carefully and avoid brands with higher amounts of sugar and carbohydrate.

L-glutamine for Building Muscle and Immune Support

L-glutamine is one of the twenty most common amino acids found in protein. It is known as a "conditionally essential" amino acid because there are times when the body cannot produce enough of it to meet its needs and must get additional L-glutamine from outside sources, such as food or supplements. This substance is important for protein synthesis, muscle function and repair, digestive efficiency, and maintaining a healthy immune system.

When you are engaged in a high-intensity workout program, L-glutamine supplementation becomes essential. The reason for this is that muscle tissue contains most of the body's L-glutamine stores, and stress, (exercise) breaks down muscle, releasing glutamine.

Glutamine depletion has a significant effect on the immune system. A study published in *Medicine and Science in Sports and Exercise* states that people develop a window of low immune function and vulnerability to disease following a session of exhaustive high-intensity training. According to this article, taking L-glutamine following HIT not only stimulates immune function but decreases inflammation and protects muscle cells from the damage induced by workout stress.

I recommend taking 5 grams of L-glutamine mixed with water or juice immediately following your workout to support immune function, help with the repair and recovery of your muscle tissue, and aid in the building of more lean muscle.

Maltodextrin

The last member of the Supersynergistic Four is maltodextrin. Maltodextrin comes in either powder form or a liquid drink such as Carboplex. It is an ideal type of carbohydrate to mix with creatine monohydrate and whey before your workout and with your whey protein shake after your workout. Maltodextrin is a very concentrated carbohydrate, pure energy that the cells in your body can draw upon during a workout. In fact, one cup of a maltodextrin drink such as Carboplex packs as much of an energy punch as six plates of whole-wheat pasta!

The advantage of maltodextrin over other types of carbohydrate such as sucrose, dextrose, or glucose is that it is absorbed more efficiently by the body and can be given in a relatively large dose without fear of gastric distress. Maltodextrin is also tasteless, which allows it to be blended with all drinks and foods.

Maltodextrin will not only give you energy *during* a workout, it can also be used to accelerate the recovery process following a workout or strenuous activity. Taken sixty to thirty minutes before the workout in combination with whey protein, it helps prevent muscle loss during exercise. Taken after exercise mixed with whey protein, maltodextrin will slowly stabilize your blood sugar level. This releases the hormone insulin, which drives the protein and carbohydrate into your muscle cells to enhance the anabolic state.

Please note that maltodextrin is not recommended for diabetics or people with hypoglycemia, obesity, or other disorders. If you have any of these conditions, it is important to get your doctor's approval before using this product.

Always Combine Maltodextrin and Whey Protein

You will notice in the supplementation schedule that I ask you to take malto-dextrin and whey protein *together* before and after your workout. When your goal is to increase lean muscle, this is the best supplementation strategy. Research has shown that an easily digestible "fast" protein such as whey and a high-quality carbohydrate such as maltodextrin work exponentially better together. A study published in *Medicine and Science in Sports and Exercise* reported: "Consumption of both protein and carbohydrate results in even greater effects on protein balance. Protein synthesis was stimulated 400 percent above pre-exercise values when a protein and carbohydrate supplement was consumed [soon] after a bout of resistance exercise."

Another study published in the *International Journal of Sport Nutrition and Exercise Metabolism* reported that "the response to amino acids [whey protein powder] alone was larger than the response to carbohydrate alone, even though the carbohydrate drink was of greater caloric value than the amino acid drink. The results of the present study support the notion that the addition of amino acids or protein to carbohydrate has an effect on muscle amino acid metabolism beyond the caloric value. . . . Thus, the addition of protein to an amino acid carbohydrate mixture prolongs the anabolic response." In other words, whey and maltodextrin taken together are an extremely efficient muscle-building duo.

However, this article goes on to state that this mixture of protein and carbs was most effective when ingested immediately after exercise. The researchers also state that there is still significant benefit if these proteins and carbs are ingested up to two hours after exercise. As we saw above, that's the window of greatest effectiveness.

Multivitamins and Antioxidants: Rounding Out the Supersynergistic Team

I would like you to add two more components to your performance nutrition supplementation program: a good multivitamin and a specific spectrum of antioxidants.

Just as most people really do not know how to take substances such as crea-tine monohydrate and maltodextrin, they do not understand the true value of vitamins, minerals, and antioxidants taken in tandem with a high-performance workout. Nor do they understand when to take vitamins to get the most value from them.

Multivitamin and Mineral Supplements

When you are involved in a high-intensity training program, it is important to take a high-quality multivitamin and mineral supplement to help increase your body's metabolic efficiency and support muscle repair and growth during your recovery periods between workouts. Vitamins also help promote general health and support a stronger immune system. When buying a multivitamin/mineral supplement, do not skimp on price since high-quality, nonsynthetic ingredients come at a higher cost. Many cheap brands of vitamins contain fillers, which may cause an allergic reaction in sensitive individuals.

Always read the label to see what you are getting. Many products provide a wide spectrum of nutrients, but I suggest taking one that includes the following:

Nutrient	Amount
Vitamin A (as beta carotene)	10,000 IU
Vitamin C (as ascorbic acid)	600 milligrams
Vitamin D	400 IU
Vitamin E	200 IU
Vitamin K	60 mcg
Thiamin	60 milligrams
Riboflavin	30 milligrams
Niacin	60 milligrams
Vitamin B_6	60 milligrams
Folic acid	800 mcg
Vitamin B_{12}	800 mcg
Biotin	600 mcg
Pantothenic acid	100 milligrams
Calcium (as calcium carbonate and calcium citrate)	500–1,000 milligrams
Iron	18 milligrams
Iodine	300 mcg
Magnesium (aspartate or glycenate)	200 and 300 milligrams
Zinc (mono-methionine)	15 milligrams
Selenium	100 mcg
Copper	1.5 milligrams
Manganese	15 milligrams
Chromium (as chromium picolinate)	200 mcg
Molybdenum	25 mcg
Boron	3 milligrams

I take the vitamins formulated by Dr. Michael Murray. They are made by a highly respected company called Natural Factors and come in special formulations for men and women. Other leading companies that make excellent multivitamin and mineral supplements are Enzymatic Therapy, NOW, Solaray, and Solgar. The staff at your local health food store will be able to assist you in picking a good brand.

When doing an HIT workout, the ideal way to take your vitamins is half a dose with breakfast and half a dose with your evening meal to avoid the "washout effect," where the water-soluble vitamins tend to be excreted by the body as the day wears on. However, if you have a vitamin that is a single-dose capsule, then take the entire dose at breakfast or with the meal before your HIT workout.

Antioxidants: Protection from Oxidative Stress

In the past, researchers established that aerobic (endurance) exercises such as running or bicycling caused oxidative stress, which resulted in damage to cellular proteins, lipids, and nucleic acids in the body. Recent studies, including one published by the Canadian Society for Exercise Physiology, found that anaerobic exercise (short bursts of intense exercise and strength training) also cause significant oxidative stress.

As a high-intensity anaerobic training program, the Lean and Hard Workout causes the body to produce a higher-than-normal level of free radicals (the factors that cause oxidative stress). For this reason, it is important to take specific doses of antioxidants to neutralize these substances before they can cause harm to your body.

The best time to take antioxidants is after your workout with a whey protein and glucose polymer shake or with your next meal. The reason for this is that free radical damage is greatest following exercise.

Be sure to check with your doctor to see if you are taking other medications that might conflict with specific antioxidants.

Free Radicals and Antioxidants

Let's take a quick look at what free radicals are, what they do, and how antioxidants work to counteract their effects on the atoms that make up our cells.

The most important factor that determines the chemical behavior of an atom is the number of electrons in its outer shell. An atom that has a full outer shell tends not to enter into chemical reactions and become inert (stable). Because atoms are designed to seek a state of maximum stability, they will try to fill their outer shells to their proper carrying capacity by gaining or losing electrons. One of the ways they accomplish this is to share electrons with other atoms by bonding with them.

Normally, bonds don't form in a way that leaves a molecule with an odd, unpaired electron. But when a weak bond splits, free radicals are formed. Free radicals are very unstable atoms that react quickly with other compounds, trying to capture the electron they need to gain stability. Generally, free radicals attack the nearest stable molecule, stealing its electron. When the attacked molecule loses its electron, it becomes a free radical itself, beginning a chain reaction. Once this process starts, it can cascade, resulting in the disruption of the living cell. The formation of free radicals is known as oxidative stress.

There are many reasons that free radicals form in the body. Some free radicals arise normally during metabolism. Sometimes the cells of the body's immune system purposefully create them to neutralize viruses and bacteria. Environmental factors such as pollution, radiation, cigarette smoke, and herbicides can also create free radicals. And, of course, all types of exercise create free radicals.

The body can usually handle free radicals, but if antioxidants aren't available or the production of free radicals passes a certain threshold, damage from oxidative stress can occur. It is important to protect and repair the body by taking antioxidants because free radical damage can cause problems such as heart disease, cancer, and insulin resistance. This damage continues to accumulate with age.

The solution is to take antioxidants, which neutralize free radicals by donating one of their own electrons, ending the electron-stealing chain reaction. Antioxidants themselves don't become free radicals when they donate an electron because they are stable in either form. They act as scavengers, helping to prevent cell and tissue damage that could lead to cellular damage and disease.

Most people are familiar with antioxidants such as vitamin C, vitamin E, and selenium. But there are other important ones that I recommend to my clients. Below are the antioxidants recommended for those involved in HIT and the some of the benefits they have for your overall health.

Since it cannot be guaranteed that your multivitamin/mineral supplement will be giving you the antioxidant dosage that I recommend, I suggest that you read the label and then adjust your daily intake by taking additional doses (as recommended by your physician). Also, check with your doctor to make sure that you are not taking any medications with which these antioxidants might interfere.

Vitamin C is the most abundant water-soluble antioxidant in the body. It is important for the synthesis of neurotransmitters—hormones that act as natural steroids—and carnitine; the conversion of cholesterol to bile; and the formation of the collagen in connective tissue. Vitamin C strengthens the immune system and helps to reduce your risk of various types of cancer and cardiovascular disease. It also has the ability to regenerate vitamin E. The recommended daily dosage for someone performing HIT is 500 to 1,000 milligrams. A recent study published in the *International Journal of Sports Nutrition and Exercise Metabolism* showed that "two weeks of [this amount of] vitamin C supplementation can partially protect against exercise induced oxidative stress in humans."

Vitamin E is a fat-soluable vitamin that also supports healthy immune function. It prevents brain cell death and may help prevent some forms of cancer.

Vitamin E is present in the lipids of cell membranes and in circulating low-density lipoproteins. When free radicals are produced as the by-products of metabolic processes and exposure to environmental pollutants, vitamin E neutralizes them. This antioxidant also helps to prevent damage to DNA that can lead to cell mutations. The recommended daily dosage for someone performing HIT is 200 IU, with medical approval if you currently suffer from heart disease. Preferably your vitamin E should be a blend of mixed tocopherols.

Selenium activates the antioxidant enzyme glutathione peroxidase, which protects red blood cells, cell membranes, and subcellular components against the oxidation caused by exercise, which can result in cell death. Selenium prolongs cell strength and cell life. The recommended daily dosage for someone performing HIT is 50 to 200 micrograms.

Zinc is an essential cofactor for many metabolic processes in the body requiring enzymes and plays an important part of strengthening the immune system. Zinc is important because people become increasingly prone to zinc deficiency as they age, which manifests as poor wound healing, poor hormonal balance, low levels of testosterone, and weakened immune function. The daily recommended dosage for someone performing HIT is 15 to 40 milligrams of zinc. Excessive zinc intake can interfere with copper absorption, so make sure not to overdo this mineral. Check with your physician for your optimum intake and type, as well as any possible medical conflicts.

Alpha lipoic acid is a powerful antioxidant that is both water and fat soluble. When compared to other antioxidants, it is even more potent than the well-known vitamins C and E. Alpha lipoic acid recycles both C and E, enhancing energy production at the cellular level and mimicking the important hormone insulin. Alpha lipoic acid may be useful in preventing and treating many disease such as diabetes. The daily recommended dosage of alpha lipoic acid for someone performing HIT is 100 milligrams. If you are hypoglycemic, diabetic, or currently under medical care, check with your physician for the proper amounts relative to any contraindications with your current medications.

Grape seed extract improves circulation and reduces pain and edema. A champion free-radical scavenger, it protects the capillary system. Grape seed has been used in the treatment of macular degeneration and works to optimize the function of other antioxidants such as vitamin C, vitamin E, and beta carotene. The daily recommended dosage for someone performing HIT is 50 milligrams.

Coenzyme Q10 is a powerful antioxidant that improves metabolic efficiency and endurance when taken before an exercise session, helps to decrease insulin resistance, and doubles your body's ability to eliminate metabolic toxins. Taking this supplement with a snack containing fat, such as a small handful of nuts or a tablespoon of peanut butter, will help your body to absorb it.

There has been extensive research in the United States and Japan regarding the treatment of cardiovascular disease with coenzyme Q10. Taking this supplement can help to keep your heart healthy. Since this supplement enhances immune function, it could also be used to decrease one's risk of cancer, particularly breast cancer. The recommended daily dosage for someone performing HIT is 50 milligrams for women and 100 milligrams for men, with physician approval.

Acetyl L-carnitine affects the mitochondria in the muscles that chew up energy. This amino acid improves muscle function and the muscles' ability to use fatty acids more efficiently. The recommended daily dose of acetyl L-carnatine is 500 milligrams for women and 1,000 milligrams for men, with physician approval.

Again, always remember to check and see how much of these antioxidants you are already receiving in your daily multiple vitamin and adjust the dosage accordingly.

Now that you've seen how all of the performance nutrition supplements work together, let's take a look at the Lean and Hard Performance Nutrition Supplementation Protocol, which will serve as your daily guide.

7

The Lean and Hard Nutrition Supplementation Schedule

The timing of when you take your supplements has everything to do with how much energy you have for your workout, how quickly you recover, and how much muscle you build. That's why it is important to take all of your supplements on schedule. The quality of the supplements you choose and the amount you take are also important. A recent article in *Medicine and Science in Sports and Exercise* states: "Quantity, quality, and timing of dietary intake around the workout influence nutrient and hormone availability at specific receptors on target tissues (i.e., skeletal muscle)."

Now that I have explained to you why I am asking you to supplement with creatine, whey protein, maltodextrin, L-glutamine, multivitamins and minerals, and antioxidants in support of your high-intensity Lean and Hard Workout, here is a day-by-day guide of when to take them and how much to take.

Again, make sure that you consult with your physician first to make sure that you have his or her approval for following this supplementation schedule.

The Schedule for Multivitamin/Mineral Supplements and Antioxidants

Multivitamin/Mineral Supplements: Take half a dose with breakfast and half a dose with dinner, five days a week. Take two days off. Make sure you always take vitamins and minerals on the days you are working out.

Antioxidants: Take them with your postworkout meal. For example, if you work out in the morning, take your antioxidants with your lunch. If you work out after work, take them with your evening meal. If you work out after your evening meal, take your antioxidants with your final snack of the day. Again, take two days off, making sure that you always take antioxidants on the days you are working out.

I ask you to take these supplements only five days a week because your body may become accustomed to them after a while and you won't get the same effect.

The exception would be if your physician suggests changing the protocol, such as asking you to take vitamins, minerals, and antioxidants daily or not at all.

Performance Nutrition Supplement Protocol: Creatine Monohydrate, Whey Protein Powder, L-Glutamine, and Maltodextrin

How Much Is a Serving?

When I say to take half or one serving of a supplement, I mean the following:

- Creatine monohydrate: ½ serving = 2½ g (½ tsp.); 1 serving = 5 g (1 tsp.)
- Whey protein: ½ serving = 10 g (½ of the scoop that comes in the canister); 1 serving = 20 g (a full scoop)
- Maltodextrin: ½ serving = ¼ cup (27 g); 1 serving = ½ cup (54.5 g)
- L-glutamine: ½ serving = 2½ g (½ tsp.); 1 serving = 5 g (1 tsp.)

When to Take the Supplements

As we have seen, the *timing* of when you take each supplement is extremely important to the success of your workout. The more closely you follow the suggested schedule, the more energy you will have for each HIT session and the more muscle you will build.

The preworkout, postworkout, and presleep supplements may be mixed together in the designated amounts in the same beverage.

Preworkout:	Take 60 to 30 minutes before workout. Mix all supplements with plain water or juice.
During workout:	Have your favorite sports drink.
Postworkout:	Preferably take immediately after workout, but *not more* than 120 minutes following workout. Mix all supplements with water, juice, or low-fat milk.
Before dinner:	Mix with water, juice, or low-fat milk.
Presleep:	Take immediately before sleep. Mix with water or juice.

WEEK 1

Monday

Before breakfast:	1 serving creatine monohydrate
Preworkout:	1 serving creatine monohydrate
	½ serving whey protein
	½ serving maltodextrin
During workout:	Your favorite sports drink
Postworkout:	1 serving creatine monohydrate
	1 serving whey protein
	1 serving maltodextrin
	1 serving L-glutamine
Before dinner:	1 serving creatine monohydrate
Presleep:	½ serving whey protein
	½ serving maltodextrin

Tuesday

Before breakfast:	1 serving creatine monohydrate
Preworkout:	1 serving creatine monohydrate
	½ serving whey protein
	½ serving maltodextrin
During workout:	Your favorite sports drink

Postworkout:	1 serving creatine monohydrate
	1 serving whey protein
	1 serving maltodextrin
	1 serving L-glutamine
Before dinner:	1 serving creatine monohydrate
Presleep:	½ serving whey protein
	½ serving maltodextrin

Wednesday (Optional Cardiovascular Workout Day)

Before breakfast:	1 serving creatine monohydrate
Preworkout:	1 serving creatine monohydrate
	½ serving whey protein
	½ serving maltodextrin
During workout:	Your favorite sports drink
Postworkout:	1 serving creatine monohydrate
	1 serving whey protein
	1 serving maltodextrin
	1 serving L-glutamine
Before dinner:	1 serving creatine monohydrate

If this is a nonworkout day, take only the creatine monohydrate as:

	1 serving prebreakfast
	1 serving prelunch
	1 serving predinner
	1 serving presleep

Thursday

Preworkout:	1 serving creatine monohydrate
	½ serving whey protein
	½ serving maltodextrin
During workout:	Your favorite sports drink
Postworkout:	1 serving whey protein
	1 serving maltodextrin
	1 serving L-glutamine

Presleep:	½ serving whey protein
	½ serving maltodextrin

Friday

Preworkout:	1 serving creatine monohydrate
	½ serving whey protein
	½ serving maltodextrin
During workout:	Your favorite sports drink
Postworkout:	1 serving whey protein
	1 serving maltodextrin
	1 serving L-glutamine
Presleep:	½ serving whey protein
	½ serving maltodextrin

Saturday

No supplementation unless you make this your optional cardio day. In that case, follow the Wednesday weeks 2, 3, and 4 supplementation schedule.

Sunday

No supplementation.

Weeks 2, 3, and 4

Monday and Thursday

Preworkout:	1 serving creatine monohydrate
	½ serving whey protein
	½ serving maltodextrin
During workout:	Your favorite sports drink
Postworkout:	1 serving whey protein
	1 serving maltodextrin
	1 serving L-glutamine
Presleep:	½ serving whey protein
	½ serving maltodextrin

Tuesday and Friday

Preworkout:	1 serving creatine monohydrate
	½ serving whey protein
	½ serving maltodextrin
During workout:	Your favorite sports drink
Postworkout:	1 serving whey protein
	1 serving maltodextrin
	1 serving L-glutamine
Presleep:	½ serving whey protein
	½ serving maltodextrin

Wednesday (Optional Cardiovascular Workout Day)

Preworkout:	½ serving creatine monohydrate
	½ serving whey protein
	½ serving maltodextrin
During workout:	Your favorite sports drink
Postworkout:	1 serving whey protein
	1 serving maltodextrin
	1 serving L-glutamine

If this is a nonworkout day, take no supplementation.

Saturday

No supplementation unless you make this your optional cardio day. In that case, follow the Wednesday weeks 2, 3, and 4 supplementation schedule.

Sunday

No supplementation.

Week 5

Monday, Tuesday, Thursday, and Friday

Preworkout:	1 serving creatine monohydrate
	½ serving whey protein
	½ serving maltodextrin
During workout:	Your favorite sports drink

Postworkout: 1 serving whey protein

1 serving maltodextrin

1 serving L-glutamine

Presleep: ½ serving whey protein

½ serving maltodextrin

Wednesday (Optional Cardiovascular Workout Day)

Preworkout: 1 serving creatine monohydrate

½ serving whey protein

½ serving maltodextrin

During workout: Your favorite sports drink

Postworkout: 1 serving whey protein

1 serving maltodextrin

1 serving L-glutamine

If this is a nonworkout day, take no supplementation.

Saturday

No supplementation unless you make this your optional cardio day. In that case, follow the Wednesday weeks 2, 3, and 4 supplementation schedule.

Sunday

No supplementation.

Week 6

Monday and Thursday

Preworkout: 1 serving creatine monohydrate

½ serving whey protein

½ serving maltodextrin

During workout: Your favorite sports drink

Postworkout: 1 serving whey protein

1 serving maltodextrin

1 serving L-glutamine

Presleep: ½ serving whey protein

½ serving maltodextrin

Tuesday and Friday

Preworkout:	1 serving creatine monohydrate
	½ serving whey protein
	½ serving maltodextrin
During workout:	Your favorite sports drink
Postworkout:	1 serving whey protein
	1 serving maltodextrin
	1 serving L-glutamine
Presleep:	½ serving whey protein
	½ serving maltodextrin

Wednesday (Optional Cardiovascular Workout Day)

Preworkout:	½ serving creatine monohydrate
	½ serving whey protein
	½ serving maltodextrin
During workout:	Your favorite sports drink
Postworkout:	1 serving whey protein
	1 serving maltodextrin
	1 serving L-glutamine

If this is a nonworkout day, take no supplementation.

Saturday

No supplementation unless you make this your optional cardio day. In that case, follow the Wednesday weeks 2, 3, and 4 supplementation schedule.

Sunday

No supplementation.

Maintenance Schedule

At this point, your physician must approve continued use of the protocol, especially with respect to creatine monohydrate.

Workout Day

During workout:	Your favorite sports drink

Postworkout:	½ serving creatine monohydrate
	1 serving whey protein
	1 serving maltodextrin
	1 serving L-glutamine
Presleep:	½ serving whey protein
(If you have had	½ serving maltodextrin
two consecutive	
high-intensity	
workout days)	

Nonworkout Day

No supplementation

PART THREE

The Lean and Hard High-Intensity Workout

8

Managing Intensity

Understand Your Body's Energy and Fuel Systems

There is a saying in AA and other recovery programs: "The system works if you work it, so work it, you're worth it." The same can be said for the Lean and Hard Program. You will get as much out of it as you put into it. If you follow the guidelines for the exercise program, the food program, and the performance nutrition supplementation schedule as described, you will be guaranteed to see results in the amount of lean muscle that you gain.

After twenty-five years of working with over three thousand professional athletes, I know the importance of learning how to efficiently use the body's energy systems to optimize muscle repair and growth.

This chapter shows how the body's three energy systems relate to your workout and why you can't just do the exercises haphazardly or mix them up, doing half of Monday's running with Tuesday's weight lifting. The more informed you are about how your body uses energy, the greater your ability to get the most muscle-building results from your time investment.

The Three Energy Systems

Many people associate being "in shape" with cardiovascular fitness, the optimum development of the heart/lung system. Although heart/lung function is a very important component of fitness, a high-intensity workout that builds strength and power does not depend primarily upon the cardiovascular system but upon other energy systems in the body.

The body has three energy systems:

1. The ATP-CP (adenosine triphosphate and creatine phosphate) system, which is responsible for explosive power in activities lasting between 8 and 10 seconds.

2. The lactic acid system, which comes into play in activities lasting up to 90 seconds.

3. The aerobic system, which works in the presence of oxygen, and kicks in after 3 minutes of continuous activity. The body uses this energy system during activities such as endurance cycling or jogging.

The explosive or high-powered exercises I am asking you to perform during your Lean and Hard Warm-Ups and Workout require *rapid* energy production in the body. For this reason, you will be learning how to efficiently use the first and second energy systems: the ATP-CP and lactic acid systems.

During a high-intensity workout, your goal is to achieve a level of performance that will enable you to build the greatest amount of lean muscle for the amount of time spent. Attaining this level of performance depends upon efficient production, use, and control of energy in the body, enabling you to get the most out of your ATP-CP and lactic acid systems during your workout.

When the energy intake (specific type of fuel) does not match the type and level of activity, an energy deficit occurs, and your muscle and liver glycogen stores will dwindle.

That is why it is vitally important for you to faithfully take your supplements before, during, and after your workout. If you fail to do so, you may "run out of gas," making you tire more easily and causing your body to break down muscle tissue for fuel. When you have all the raw materials on hand to keep your energy engine running like a fine race car, you will exercise more effectively and build lean muscle more efficiently.

Let's take a closer look at each of the three energy systems and how they function during your workout.

The ATP-CP System: The Body's Powerhouse

All living things require a constant supply of energy to function. This energy is used in all the processes that keep the organism alive. Some of these processes occur continually, such as the metabolism of foods. Others occur only at certain times, such as during the contraction of a muscle.

Before the energy stored in our cells can be used during a high-intensity workout, it must first be transformed into a form that the body can handle easily. The special storehouses of energy are the molecules known as CP, creatine phosphate, and adenosine triphosphate, or ATP for short.

ATP is the primary energy source for every cell in your body, including those found in your muscle fibers. This energy is used not only to fuel muscular contractions when you work out but to repair cells once the workout is finished. Remember, a high-intensity workout does not build muscle, it breaks it down, creating the potential for greater muscularity. It is what you eat and drink following a workout to repair muscle that makes the muscle get larger. The efficiency with which your body can repair muscle fibers is the most vital aspect of getting lean and hard.

The "triphosphate" in ATP simply refers to three phosphate molecules. When you perform high-intensity exercise, an enzymatic reaction in your body removes one of the phosphate molecules from ATP, releasing a very high level of energy and producing adenosine *di*phosphate. Without this energy, your muscles would be unable to contract and your body would be unable to build proteins.

When you are resting during a workout or recovering afterward, the reverse reaction is taking place—your body is reconfiguring each ATP molecule by reattaching a phosphate molecule taken from the CP (creatine phosphate) molecules in your muscle tissue. While CP occurs naturally in the body, there is not enough available to supply the needs of frequent high-intensity training sessions such as the Lean and Hard Workout.

While you could *complete* the exercises without taking the performance supplementation, once your CP stores were exhausted, your body could begin using the protein in your muscles as fuel. This would go against the purpose of the program in this book, which is to *spare* lean muscle during the workout and to *build* muscle during the recovery periods after the HIT session.

When Is the ATP-CP System Activated During Your Lean and Hard Workout?

The body activates the ATP-CP system during short bouts (up to 15 seconds) of powerful, explosive activities such as a 40-yard dash. Since the time element of these activities is so short, the body doesn't have time to accumulate high levels of lactic acid. That is why this energy system is also referred to as the "alactic" system.

Exercises requiring short intense bursts of energy require adequate recovery; for example, a 5-second sprint followed by 20 to 50 seconds of rest. However, as your body becomes more accustomed to brief, explosive episodes of exercise during workouts, the recovery periods in between events will lessen somewhat.

Monday and Thursday of the Lean and Hard Workout will use the ATP-PC system.

Here is a brief summary of the mechanism of the ATP and PC energy system.

- ATP is broken down to make the muscle contract. The result is ADP (adenosine diphosphate).

- A phosphate molecule is taken from the CP (creatine phosphate) reservoir in your cells and attached to ADP to re-create an ATP molecule.
- The process starts over again when your ATP molecules—the special storehouse in your cells—lose a phosphate molecule once again, releasing an explosive amount of energy to help your muscles contract or repair themselves following the workout.
- Since the amount of CP your body stores runs out after 8 to 10 seconds of intense activity, you can see why supplementing with creatine monohydrate extends your ATP production.
- The ATP-CP system requires 3 to 5 minutes for restoration.

The Lactic Acid System

When you perform exercises involving speed, endurance, or weight lifting—events lasting between 30 and 90 seconds—you will be using your lactic acid system. The slight irritation caused by the accumulation of lactic acid in the tissues is one of the stimulating mechanisms that causes the body to create greater lean muscle mass by building itself back up.

The energy that powers the lactic acid system comes from the complex carbohydrate known as glycogen, stored in your muscles and your liver. Your muscle cell first breaks down the glycogen into glucose, then metabolizes it to make ATP. This is known as anaerobic metabolism because it completes this process without the use of oxygen.

This system provides more total energy than the CP (creatine phosphate) mechanism. That's why it lasts longer before rest is needed—up to 90 seconds in the conditioned athlete.

Because you will be using up glycogen (carbohydrate) stores in your muscles when using your lactic acid system, you should ingest glucose polymers before, during, and after your workout and include an appropriate amount of complex carbohydrates in your high-performance food program.

If you neglect to take the high-performance nutritional supplements required to restore your lactic acid system following high-intensity training, your body will not have sufficient ATP to repair muscle tissue. The result will be little or no muscle growth following all your hard work, low energy, and a possible reduction in strength during your next workout.

You will be emphasizing the lactic acid system when doing the interval training exercises on Tuesday and Friday.

Here is a summary of how the lactic acid system works during your high-intensity workout:

- Muscle and liver glycogen is broken down to produce energy, which in turn produces ATP.
- This process can occur with or without the presence of oxygen—without

oxygen during the workout and with oxygen when you are at rest during or after the workout.

- The production of ATP without oxygen leads to the formation of lactic acid.
- An excess accumulation of lactic acid causes muscle fatigue (a burning sensation).
- This system is an excellent source of fuel for high-intensity events lasting between 30 and 90 seconds.

Following a session of high-intensity strength training, the restoration of glycogen in the liver and muscles takes time, as detailed below.

- 2 hours to restore 40 percent
- 5 hours to restore 55 percent
- 24 or more hours to restore 100 percent

The Aerobic Energy System

The third and final energy system is known as the aerobic (endurance) system, which includes any long-lasting, steady-state-type of activity done in the presence of oxygen. Examples of aerobic exercise are continuous running over distance, such as a marathon; elliptical training; and cycle training. The aerobic system uses carbohydrate, fat, and protein with oxygen to produce ATP.

Steady-state aerobic exercises have been shown to help clear the body of lactic acid and raise the fatigue threshold, so I have suggested either Wednesday or Saturday as a day for an optional cardiovascular workout, which I describe in the next chapter, or for any cardiovascular activities that you enjoy. However, this aerobic component truly is optional because the Lean and Hard Program increases the cardiovascular system an average of 31 percent using high-intensity interval training alone.

Here is an overview of how the aerobic system works:

- It requires an average of 60 to 80 seconds to start producing energy.
- It depends primarily upon carbohydrate and fat as its fuel source.
- Carbohydrate is a more efficient fuel than fat to operate the aerobic system.
- Since carbohydrate stores are limited, they must be replenished for optimal performance during an endurance event.
- Since the body's fat stores are greater than its carbohydrate stores, as aerobic training progresses, the body will use fat stores with greater efficiency.
- For most people, it takes 20 to 25 minutes of low to moderate aerobic exercise for your body to shift to effectively burning fat as its primary fuel. We are always burning a certain amount of carbohydrate and fat

during any activity. However, when an endurance activity is extended beyond a certain amount of time, there is a greater potential for fat oxidation. That's why in a weight-loss program, aerobic exercise should last a minimum of 30 minutes to ensure the burning of excess fat.

- It may take between 18 and 48 hours for the complete restoration of the aerobic energy system.

It Works If You Work It

The Lean and Hard system is not haphazard. It is all laid out for you, in a simple and easy to follow format. If you eat the right amount and kinds of calories, take the performance nutrition supplements on schedule, and do the exercises in the order they are presented for the time I suggest, your body will build lean muscle and become toned and tight.

A great example of the benefits of following the Lean and Hard guidelines can be seen in a former Navy SEAL who was part of the original study. This individual gained the highest amount of muscle, 20 pounds, and dropped his body fat percentage from 4 percent to 2 percent. While this was the *lowest* fat loss in the study, for him it was 50 percent!

He achieved this muscle gain by following the program as faithfully as he could, making sure that he ate the right foods, took all his performance nutrition supplements right on schedule, and did the exercises in the right order on the correct days.

In his words, "I am someone who is used to following orders because during my years as a Navy SEAL, when I constantly found myself in dangerous situations, my very life often depended upon following the guidelines I was given. In those days, I always trained as hard as I could because I had to give a consistently greater effort greater than the enemy.

"So, I'm sold on believing in the importance of a good system. Your program was simple and easy to follow. It gave me structure, an understanding of why you were asking me to do the exercises, and the nutrients and diet that fueled me with the energy to carry out the plan."

The more faithfully you follow the Lean and Hard exercise and performance nutrition guidelines, the more muscle you can expect to gain. It's as simple as that.

9

Lean and Hard Warm-Ups and Drills

What You Need to Know before You Begin Your High-Intensity Workout

Before you begin your Lean and Hard Workout, you need to be checked out by your doctor. Then you need to become familiar with the terminology that will be used in the exercise program. This includes learning what it means to monitor your heart rate at different levels of intensity, becoming familiar with your rate of perceived exertion (RPE), learning the names and definitions of certain types of exercises and drills, and familiarizing yourself with the warm-up. First, let's take a look at the kinds of exercise you will be doing.

The Four Basic Kinds of High-Intesity Training Exercise

There are four basic types of exercise in the Lean and Hard Workout:

1. Anaerobic, or interval training, a form of exercise that alternates short spurts of high-intensity effort with short periods of lesser intensity (active rest)

2. Core exercises to strengthen and stabilize the lower back and abdominal area of the body

3. Strength building, which includes dumbbell and free-weight routines and working out on machines at the gym

4. Optional aerobic exercises, which include activities done at a steady state of exertion, such as walking, running, elliptical training, or riding a bicycle

Remember to have a complete physical exam by your physician before beginning a new exercise routine.

Interval Training and Your High-Intensity Training Workout

Except for the performance stretching routines, which warm up the specific muscle groups you will use that day, the Lean and Hard Workout is based completely on interval training (anaerobic activities). The workout guidelines in this chapter will show you how to perform speed improvement drills, core exercises, and strength-building exercises anaerobically (at high-intensity intervals) as opposed to aerobically (at a steady state).

Studies have shown that interval training is the most effective form of exercise for improving body composition and building lean muscle. For example, let's take a look at a recent study on interval training published in the *Journal of Metabolism*. The first test group performed aerobic exercise at moderate intensity for 20 minutes at a time. The second group performed high-intensity interval training for shorter periods of time. At the end of three months, the second group had lost nine times more fat than the first group and gained more lean muscle.

Managing Intensity and Fatigue: Creating a Positive Energy Balance

Once you understand *why* I am asking you to do high-intensity interval training, the next step is to define what "high-intensity" means for you. If you have ever worked out in a gym for any length of time, you've probably witnessed a scenario like the following.

An out-of-shape individual, let's call him Mark, decides to join his local gym to build muscle and trim some fat. However, Mark doesn't have a clear idea of how to exercise effectively and doesn't seek the assistance of a trainer who could help him understand what low, medium, and high levels of exercise intensity mean for him. Mark goes from machine to machine, piling on the weight and exercising to the point of exhaustion. This isn't a smart way to begin a new workout regimen for many reasons. First, Mark is trying to eat as few calories as possible so that he can "get lean and lose fat." Ironically, because his body lacks sufficient fuel to efficiently repair and build lean muscle, and because he does not know how to manage his energy efficiently to offset the fatigue of training, he isn't seeing results. If anything, he finds himself getting softer.

Frustrated, he pushes himself harder and harder, always trying for a "maximum" level of intensity, but instead getting a maximum level of fatigue that makes it hard for him to finish each set. Eventually, he either injures himself or gives up in frustration. And that is the last we see of Mark.

What Mark really needs to do to manage fatigue and build muscle is to maintain a *positive energy balance*. In other words, he has to ingest sufficient protein, carbohydrate, fat, and performance nutrition supplementation to support his high-intensity workout and help him to make lean tissue gains. And he must make sure that he is eating the *right* kinds of nutrients, especially sufficient good carbs and lean protein.

What Does High Intensity Mean for You?

To get the optimum results from any high-performance training program, you must learn how to manage your energy level to delay fatigue. Since each person is unique in his or her level of fitness, the key element to fatigue management is training at the proper level of intensity *for you*.

There are two ways to manage your level of intensity. The first method is to learn to calculate the heart rate zones that represent your minimum, moderate, and maximum efforts. The second method is to establish your rate of perceived exertion (RPE), which can be calculated by using the instinctive intensity training (IIT) scale I include later in this chapter (see page 126).

I will be asking you to use one or the other of these methods, depending on what sort of exercise you are performing. For exercises of shorter duration, such as the drills and short sprints, I will be asking you to use a prescribed level of RPE because there will not be enough time for your heart rate to rise to a "target" level. When you are performing exercises of longer duration, such as shuttles, I will be asking you to use your target heart rate, since there will be sufficient time for your heart rate to rise into your target zone.

I have clearly indicated which method to use for which exercise in chapter 11, "The Lean and Hard Workout," which provides a detailed overview of your workout, day by day and exercise by exercise.

Intensity: Reach Your Target Training Zone

In order to maximize the results you get from your Lean and Hard Workout, you will want to do each of the drills and exercises in the Daily Workout Guide (starting on page 174) at the proper level of intensity, according to your gender, age, and fitness level. For this reason, it is important to monitor your heart rate during some phases of your workout. The instructions below will teach you how to do the following:

- Measure your heart rate by correctly taking your pulse, whether at rest or during a workout
- Measure your resting heart rate
- Calculate your target heart rate zones for mild, moderate, and vigorous levels of activity

Keep in mind that certain types of medication may alter your heart rate response to exercise, so seek your doctor's advice regarding exercise intensity relative to the effects of your medication.

The Correct Way to Take Your Pulse Manually

1. Use your middle and index fingers to take your pulse.
2. There are two locations you can use: on the neck below the chin next to the Adam's apple, or on the thumb side of the inside of the wrist.
3. Hold the index and middle fingers together against one of the two sites. (The neck is the easiest during exercise.) Count for fifteen seconds and multiply that number by four to establish your heart rate per minute.
4. Do not press too hard, especially when taking a neck pulse. Excessive pressure can reduce blood flow and cause the heart to slow down.

When working out, you may prefer to purchase a pulse rate monitor, which you can wear on your wrist, giving you a continual status of your heart rate throughout the training session. I always wear a pulse rate monitor and encourage the athletes with whom I work to do the same.

Once you have learned how to correctly take your pulse, the next step will be to determine your resting heart rate (RHR), which is defined as the number of beats per minute at complete rest.

Calculating Your Resting Heart Rate

1. First, you will need to take your morning resting heart rate. To do this, take your pulse immediately upon wakening and before you get out of bed. If your bladder is full, you didn't sleep well, or you're feeling stressed, your RHR may be slightly elevated.
2. Next take your evening resting heart rate. Take a good book to bed or listen to soothing music. After lying in a prone position for ten to twenty minutes, take your pulse.
3. Take both of these measurements for seven days and average them. This is your current RHR.
4. After two weeks of exercise, recheck your RHR.

Lean and Hard Warm-Ups and Drills   125

Calculating Your Target Heart Rate

The next step is to calculate your target heart rate (THR), which will enable you to do the drills and exercises at the appropriate level of intensity for your age and gender. The formula you will use below is called the Karvonen formula.

There are four activity levels that you will be using while performing the Lean and Hard Drills and Workout. They are calculated based upon percentage of your maximum effort. Please note that no individual, even a professional athlete, ever trains at 100 percent effort all the time. The only result would be a quick descent into fatigue and physical burnout. An effort level of 80 percent is considered to be the highest level of intensity you should attempt for optimum results.

The level of effort with which you should do each drill and exercise is clearly indicated in the Daily Workout Guide.

Level 1: Warm-up activity level   40 percent effort
Level 2: Mild activity level   60 percent effort
Level 3: Moderate activity level   70 percent effort
Level 4: Vigorous activity level   80 percent effort

If you are a man, use this formula to calculate your target heart rate:

Step 1. 220 minus your age minus your resting heart rate: ___
Step 2. Multiply this number by the activity percent level: ___
Step 3. Add this number to your resting heart rate: ___

The final number you get will be your estimated target heart rate in beats per minute (bpm) for your activity level.

If you are a woman, your formula will start with a slightly higher number:

Step 1. 230 minus your age minus your resting heart rate: ___
Step 2. Multiply this number by the percent of your activity level: ___
Step 3. Add this number to your resting heart rate: ___

The final number you get will be your estimated target heart rate in beats per minute (bpm) for your activity level.

Let's look at an example of a thirty-year-old woman with a resting heart rate of sixty beats per minute who needs to calculate her heart rate for an exercise requiring moderate effort (70 percent effort).

Step 1. 230 − 30 (age) = 200
         200 − 60 (resting heart rate) = 140
Step 2. 140 × 70 percent (.70) activity level = 98
Step 3. 98 + 60 (resting heart rate) = 158 (target heart rate for activity level)

Monitoring Your Target Heart Rate

Since your goal is to stay within your target heart rate during each set of agility drills and interval activities (sprints), you will want to monitor it off and on. Either take your pulse during the exercise or take the easier route of wearing a heart rate monitor.

If your pulse rate is much higher than your target training zone, lessen your exercise intensity by either decreasing your speed and/or increasing the recovery time between the drills or sprints. If your pulse rate is lower than your target training zone, you may want to work harder by doing just the opposite, increasing speed and/or shortening your recovery time. Should you feel any pain or prolonged discomfort, stop exercising immediately and check with your doctor.

After a while you will be able to sense when you are in your training zone by how you feel as your workout progresses. If you are breezing through the agility drills or interval sprints without any apparent exertion, you are probably below your target heart rate zone.

The Rate of Perceived Exertion: Instinctive Intensity Training

A simple and effective way to monitor your intensity level so that you get the most out of your workout is my instinctive intensity training (IIT) scale, based upon the rate of perceived exertion (RPE). Once you have checked with your doctor to make sure that there are no restrictions on your ability to exercise, go to your gym, warm up carefully, then see what you would consider to be your maximum effort. If you are overweight or have any health problems that might put you at risk, you may choose to perform this maximum effort test as part of a pulmonary stress test in the presence of your physician or a cardiologist. Your insurance may pay for this test with the appropriate diagnosis and CPT code.

Once you've identified what your maximum effort feels like, use the following scale to find the appropriate IIT level for your workout.

THE INSTINCTIVE INTENSITY TRAINING SCALE

IIT Level	Percentage of Maximum Effort	Perception
4	40	Warm-up effort
6	60	Mild effort
7	70	Moderate effort
8	80	Strong effort
9	90	Very strong effort
10	100	Maximum effort

The concept behind the IIT scale is that no one can tell you exactly how much weight you need to use or how vigorously you need to exercise. How you perceive whether an exercise is low, moderate, or high intensity is a subjective experience based upon your general level of fitness. A level of effort that seems easy for one person might present a challenge to another person, especially if he or she is deconditioned or overweightw or hasn't exercised for a while.

To find your appropriate IIT level, your rate of perceived exertion, you must learn to listen to your body. That means paying attention to a broad spectrum of physical sensations, including fatigue levels, muscle or leg pain, physical stress, and shortness of breath. For each type of exercise you do, you need to estimate how hard you need to work to achieve the desired level of intensity.

Research has shown that your perception of the amount of effort you feel you are putting into an activity is likely to agree with the actual physical measurements of that physical effort. In other words, if you feel that you are exercising moderately, measurements of things such as how fast your heart is beating would probably confirm that you are exercising at a moderate level. For example, during moderate activity you can sense that you are challenging yourself but are not yet near your limit.

In the Lean and Hard Daily Workout Guide, you will notice that I suggest monitoring your heart rate in some exercises and using the RPE in others. Each instance is clearly marked.

Rest and Recovery

Be sure to pay close attention to the periods of rest I recommend after each exercise. This time allows for the restoration of muscle energy (ATP), which is critical to making rapid gains in muscle. You won't reap the maximum benefits of this program unless you allow your body to sufficiently rest and recover as recommended. Remember, don't beat up a beat-up muscle.

The Lean and Hard drills and exercise protocol have been carefully developed so that you can successfully manage fatigue and recover your body between sets and workouts. Make sure that you adhere closely to the workout charts, the order of exercises, the intensity levels, and the number of sets and reps. Every detail of this program has been designed to not only maximize your gains but also to allow you to train harder, longer, and with less pain and fatigue than ever before.

A warm-up and a cooldown precede and follow every workout. These activities prepare the body for the workout and accelerate your recovery time. Again, follow these portions of the program very carefully. They are just as important as the strength and speed exercises.

Now let's look at the vocabulary behind each segment of the Lean and Hard Workout. This section will familiarize you with the terminology used in describing the speed-improvement drills (SIDs), buildups, and the exercises that comprise the energy management system.

Understanding Speed-Improvement Drills

Speed-improvement drills create increased flexibility in the hip area and are crucial for attaining great gains in speed. They are performed after a general warm-up of light jogging and lower body stretches. To prepare for the SIDs, mark off distances of 10, 20, and 30 yards on your track or running surface. Your Lean and Hard Daily Workout Guide gives you detailed instructions on how to do these drills. You will notice that I ask you to use the RPE when performing buildups.

Skip: Everyone knows how to do this. Alternate your legs for the total distance. Strive for height and upward drive.

Hip: Keep your body upright and maintain good running form. Exaggerate the lifting of your knees, bringing your thighs up parallel to the ground with each stride. Slightly exaggerate your arm movement as well.

Carioca: With your shoulders square, move sideways by crossing one foot over the other. Continue for the recommended distance. Then repeat facing the other way, crossing over with the opposite leg.

Butt kicks: Run the recommended distance, kicking your heels up to your buttocks in rapid succession.

Backward running: Maintain good upright body position and sprint backward. Stay low with your torso centered over your feet. Keep your feet close to the ground and pump your arms.

Quick feet: Take as many steps as possible, crossing each foot in front of the opposite ankle with quick, dynamic movements.

Stride: Move across the recommended distance by taking large strides as fast as you can. Do not break into a run. Be sure that one foot is on the ground at all times.

Power transition: Cover a 30-yard distance by skipping for 10 yards, hipping for 10 yards, and striding for 10 yards. Concentrate on making smooth transitions without stopping or losing your form.

Jumping rope: The number of times you jump in 60 seconds depends upon your level of fitness. Find your category and build up from there.

- Rookie: 100 skips in 60 seconds
- Minor league: 110 skips in 60 seconds
- Major league: 120 skips in 60 seconds

Understanding Buildups

A buildup is a medium-distance run broken into varying levels of intensity. On your track or running surface, mark off distances of 40, 80, and 120 yards.

Run the full 120 yards in the following pattern. Based on the intensity level (target heart rate or RPE) in your Daily Workout Guide, accelerate over the first 40 yards, maintain your speed for the next 40 yards, then decelerate for the final 40 yards.

Immediately walk back the full 120 yards and do another repetition, according to the workout guide.

Note: use RPE when performing buildups.

Understand the Energy Management System

These speed exercises require you to run varying distances at varying levels of intensity. Your Daily Workout Guide shows the distance, the intensity level (target heart rate or RPE), and the number of repetitions for each exercise.

Complete all repetitions and complete each distance before proceeding to the next distance and intensity level. Should you experience any pain or unusual discomfort, discontinue the drill and consult your physician.

After each run, give yourself a full recovery period by walking the distance you just ran and allowing your heart rate to return to a recovery rate of approximately 120 bpm. Be sure to adhere to the required intensity level during each repetition of the exercise.

Shorter Sprints

On some days you will be running shorter sprints. On these days I will ask you to use the RPE to monitor intensity.

Before you do your shorter sprints, mark off distances of 40, 60, and 100 yards.

- For a 40-yard sprint: Run 40 yards and walk back.
- For a 60-yard sprint: Run 60 yards and walk back.
- For a 100-yard sprint: Run 100 yards and walk back.

Longer Sprints

On some days you will be running longer sprints. On those days, instead of your RPE, you will be using your heart rate to monitor intensity. (More distance and more time allow your heart rate to increase to the required bpm. On shorter sprints there is no time to reach target heart rate zones.)

Before you begin your longer sprints, mark off distances of 100 yards and 220 yards.

- For a 100-yard sprint: Run 100 yards and walk back.
- For a 220-yard sprint: Run 220 yards and walk back.

Shuttles

Shuttles differ from sprints in that you run back the distance instead of walking it. Before you begin your shuttles, mark off distances of 5, 10, 15, and 20 yards.

- For a 60-yard shuttle: Run 5 yards and run back. Run 10 yards and run back. Run 15 yards and run back.
- For a 100-yard shuttle: Run 5 yards and run back. Run 10 yards and run back. Run 15 yards and run back. Run 20 yards and run back.

If you desire more intensity, repeat the shuttles before moving on to the next segment of your workout.

Half-Gasser

A half-gasser is a longer-distance speed drill. This is a very intense type of exercise, so you will not be performing these runs until later in the workout when you have had a chance to build up your strength and speed. The first time you will be performing a half-gasser is Week 5, Day 5 in the Daily Workout Guide.

For this speed endurance exercise, mark off 55 yards (the width of a football field). Run 55 yards, turn around, and run back at an intensity level determined by your own ability and RPE. As you improve, try to bring down this time.

Set your own time and seek to improve it based upon your recovery ability. This is true for all timed exercises. Use a time that best suits your needs and ability. Don't overdo it.

Flexibility and Stretching Exercises

Flexibility is an integral part of the program. Stretching reduces the risk of injury and minimizes muscle soreness. The following guidelines should be used for all flexibility and stretching exercises:

- Always stretch a warm muscle. If you do the general warm-up found at the beginning of each session in the Daily Workout Guide (jogging 440 yards or spending 5 minutes on a stationary bike or an elliptical machine), you will be sufficiently warmed up to begin the stretching routine.
- Stretch in a slow, controlled manner, concentrating on elongating your body and breathing into all of your stretches in a controlled and relaxed way.
- Use a slow, deep, and rhythmic breathing pattern.
- Do not bounce. Short, jerky movements give your muscles a confusing mixed message of rapid stretching and contraction.

- Never overstretch, even if your body is naturally limber.
- Never "lock" your joints or extend a muscle beyond its joint capacity. Instead, allow your knees and elbows to be slightly bent at all times (a "soft-lock" position). This will protect your joints and muscles from unnecessary wear and tear.
- If you feel pain, *stop*.

To prepare yourself for the specific exercises used in the Lean and Hard Workout, I have included three stretching routines with pictures and directions for performing them. These routines were provided by Bob and Gene Andersen from their book *Stretching*.

Stretches for Speed-Improvement Drills, Sprints, and Half-Gassers

1. Raise the tops of your shoulders toward your ears until you feel a slight tension in your neck and shoulders. Hold for 5 seconds, then relax your shoulders downward.

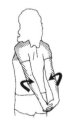

2. Interlace your fingers behind your back. Slowly turn your elbows inward while straightening your arms. Hold for 5 to 10 seconds. Do twice.

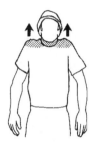

3. To stretch your calf, stand a little way from a solid support such as a wall and lean on it with your forearms, head resting on your hands. Bend one leg and place your foot on the ground in front of you, with the other leg straight behind. Slowly move your hips forward, keeping your lower back flat. Be sure to keep the heel of the straight leg on the ground, with your toes pointed straight ahead or slightly turned in. Hold an easy stretch for 10 to 15 seconds. Do not bounce. Now stretch the other leg.

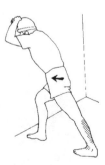

4. To stretch the quads and knees, hold the top of your *right* foot with your *left* hand and gently pull your heel toward your buttocks. The knee bends at a natural angle when you hold your foot with the opposite hand. Hold for 10 to 20 seconds for each leg. If necessary, place your other hand on a support for balance.

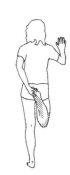

5. Stand on one foot with you knee slightly flexed and place the outside of the opposite leg just above your knee. Put one hand on the inside of your ankle and the other on your thigh. Now bend your knee a little more as you move your chest forward over the bent leg. This will test your balance. Hold a mild stretch for 10 seconds. Do both sides. This stretches the outside of the hip. Do not hold your breath.

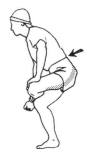

6. Assume a bent-knee position with your heels flat, toes pointed straight ahead, and feet about shoulder-width apart. Hold for 30 seconds. In this bent-knee position, you are contracting the quadriceps and relaxing the hamstrings. The primary function of the quadriceps is to straighten the leg. The basic function of the hamstrings is to bend the knee. Because these muscles have opposing actions, contracting the quadriceps will relax the hamstrings.

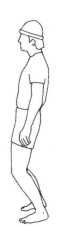

   As you hold this bent-knee position, feel the difference between the front and back of your thigh. The quadriceps should feel hard and tight, while the hamstrings should feel soft and relaxed. It's easier to stretch the hamstrings if they are first relaxed.

7. After holding the bent-knee position, stand up and then bend down again with knees slightly bent (1 inch). Let your neck, arms, and hands relax. Go to the point where you feel a slight stretch in the back of your legs. Stretch in this easy phase for 1 to 15 seconds until you are relaxed. Do not bounce, lock your knees, or overstretch.

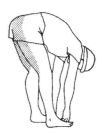

8. Move one leg forward until the knee of the forward leg is directly over the ankle. Your other knee should be resting on the ground. Place your hands on top of each other on your thigh, just above your knee. To stretch the front of your hips and thigh, straighten your arms to keep your upper body upright as your lower the front of your hip downward. This is an excellent stretch for your lower back area. Hold for 10 to 15 seconds. Repeat on the other side.

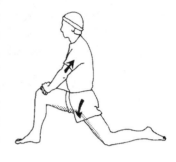

9. Start in a standing position with your knees slightly flexed to give you better balance. With your arms overhead, hold the elbow of one arm with the hand of the other arm. Gently pull your elbow behind your head as you bend from your hips to the side. Hold an easy stretch for 10 seconds. Repeat on the other side. Do not forget to breathe.

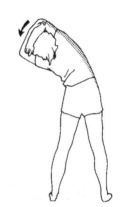

Upper Body Stretches

1. Interlace your fingers above your head. With your palms facing upward, push your arms slightly back and up. Feel the stretch in your arms, shoulders, and upper back. Hold the stretch for 15 seconds. Do not hold your breath.

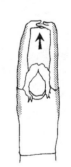

2. With your fingers interlaced behind your head, keep your elbows straight out to your sides with your upper body in a good, aligned position. Now pull your shoulder blades toward each other to create a feeling of tension through the upper back and shoulder blade area. Hold this feeling of mild tension for 4 to 5 seconds, then relax. Repeat several times.

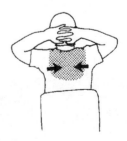

3. Start in a standing position with your knees slightly flexed. Bend your right elbow and put your arm behind your head. Hold onto your right elbow with your left hand. Keeping your knees slightly bent (about 1 inch), gently pull your elbow behind your head as you bend from your hips to the side. Keeping your knees slightly bent will give you better balance.

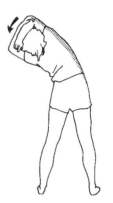

4. Hold a towel near both ends with your hands far enough apart that you can move it with straight arms up, over your head, and down behind your back with relatively free movement. Do not strain or force the stretch. Breathe slowly. Do not hold your breath.

   To increase the stretch, move your hands slightly closer together and, keeping the arms straight, repeat the movement. Move slowly and feel the stretch. Do not overstretch. If you are unable to go through the full movement of up, over, and behind while keeping your arms straight, then your hands are too close together. Move them farther apart.

   You can hold the stretch at any place during this movement. This will isolate and add more of a stretch to the muscles of that particular area. Hold for 10 to 15 seconds.

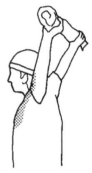

5. To stretch your shoulder and the middle of your upper back, gently pull your elbow across your chest toward your opposite shoulder. Hold for 10 seconds. Repeat on the other side.

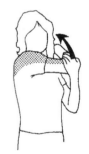

6. To stretch the side of your neck, lean your head sideways toward your left shoulder as your left hand pulls your right arm down and across, behind your back. Hold an easy stretch for 10 to 15 seconds. Repeat on the other side. Do not hold your breath.

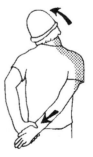

7. Interlace your fingers out in front of you at shoulder height. Turn your palms outward as you extend your arms forward to feel a stretch in your shoulders, mid-upper back, arms, hands, fingers, and wrists. Hold an easy stretch for 15 seconds, then relax and repeat.

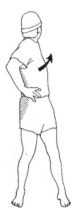

8. Start with your hands on your hips, feet pointed straight ahead, and knees slightly bent. Rotate your hips to the left as you look over your left shoulder. Hold an easy stretch for 10 seconds. Stretch each side twice. Be relaxed during this stretch and breathe easily.

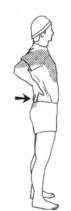

9. Standing with your knees slightly bent, place your palms on your lower back just above your hips, fingers pointing downward. Gently push your palms forward to create an extension in the lower back. Hold for 10 seconds. Repeat twice. Do not hold your breath.

Lower Body Stretches

1. To stretch your calf, stand a little way from a solid support such as a wall and lean on it with your forearms, head resting on your hands. Bend one leg and place your foot on the ground in front of you, with the other leg straight behind. Slowly move your hips forward, keeping your lower back flat. Be sure to keep the heel of the straight leg on the ground, with your toes pointed straight ahead or slightly turned in. Hold an easy stretch for 10 to 15 seconds. Do not bounce. Now stretch the other leg.

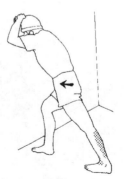

2. To stretch the quads and knees, hold the top of your *right* foot with your *left* hand and gently pull your heel toward your buttocks. The knee bends at a natural angle when you hold your foot with the opposite hand. Hold for 10 to 20 seconds for each leg. If necessary, place your other hand on a support for balance.

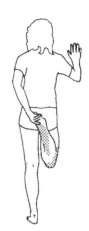

3. Assume a bent-knee position with your heels flat, toes pointed straight ahead, and feet about shoulder-width apart. Hold for 30 seconds. In this bent-knee position, you are contracting the quadriceps and relaxing the hamstrings. The primary function of the quadriceps is to straighten the leg. The basic function of the hamstrings is to bend the knee. Because these muscles have opposing actions, contracting the quadriceps will relax the hamstrings.

    As you hold this bent-knee position, feel the difference between the front and back of your thigh. The quadriceps should feel hard and tight, while the hamstrings should feel soft and relaxed. It's easier to stretch the hamstrings if they are first relaxed.

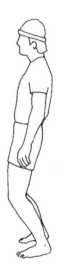

4. After holding the bent-knee position, stand up and then bend down again with knees slightly bent (1 inch). Let your neck, arms, and hands relax. Go to the point where you feel a slight stretch in the back of your legs. Stretch in this easy phase for 1 to 15 seconds until you are relaxed. Do not bounce, lock your knees, or overstretch.

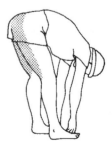

5. With your feet shoulder width apart and pointed out to about a 15-degree angle, heels on the ground, bend your knees and squat down. If you have trouble staying in this position, hold onto something for support. Hold the stretch for 10 to 20 seconds. *Be careful if you have any knee problems. If you feel pain, discontinue this stretch.*

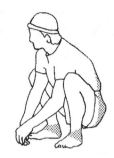

6. Move one leg forward until the knee of the forward leg is directly over the ankle. Your other knee should be resting on the ground. Without changing the position of the knee on the floor or the forward foot, lower the front of your hip downward to create an easy stretch. This stretch should be felt in the front of the hip and possibly in your hamstrings and groin. This will help relieve tension in the lower back. Hold the stretch for 20 to 30 seconds. Repeat with the other leg.

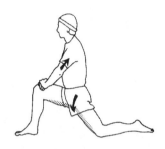

7. Start with your feet pointed straight ahead and a little more than shoulder width apart. Bend your right knee slightly and move your left hip downward toward the right knee. This gives you a stretch in your left inner thigh (left groin). Hold for 10 to 15 seconds and repeat for your right thigh.

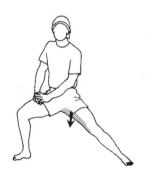

8. Start with your hands on your hips, feet pointed straight ahead, and knees slightly bent. Rotate your hips to the left as you look over your left shoulder. Hold an easy stretch for 10 seconds. Stretch each side twice. Be relaxed during this stretch and breathe easily.

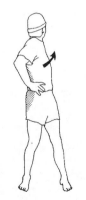

9. Standing with your knees slightly bent, place your palms on your lower back just above your hips, fingers pointing downward. Gently push your palms forward to create an extension in the lower back. Hold for 10 seconds. Repeat twice. Do not hold your breath.

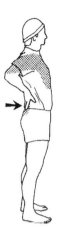

10

The Lean and Hard High-Intensity Exercises

The Lean and Hard Workout is designed to help you build lean muscle quickly and effectively through the mastery of three key factors: strength management, speed management, and fatigue management. Let's take a look at what that means to you.

Strength Management

The benefit of the Lean and Hard Workout is that it teaches you to carefully manage your strength. A strong core area (abdominals, lower back, hips, and rotators) is crucial to supporting the power of your exercise program and maximizing your performance, so you will be doing pelvic stabilizer exercises on every workout day. You will be alternating between upper and lower body core exercises every other workout. You will also be alternating between upper and lower body resistance exercises (dumbbells, free weights, and machines) in a periodized manner (increasing the sets and decreasing reps as you move through the program).

Speed Management

As you saw in the last chapter when we discussed drills, an important element of this program is the management of speed. The drills will help you to increase your speed through learning effective running mechanics, which will increase your leg strength, range of motion, and stride frequency, and improve your general conditioning. Speed-improvement drills, buildups, sprints, shuttles, and half-gassers are an integral part of your speed management program.

Fatigue Management

One of the reasons why it is so important to do the exercises exactly as they are set out in the Daily Workout Guide is the effective management of fatigue. The sequence of the exercises in this program is specifically designed with this goal in mind: to assist lactic acid clearance in order to minimize the effects of fatigue and maximize recovery.

Monday and Thursday are short sprints, which should not cause the accumulation of lactic acid (alactic), while Tuesday and Friday's longer sprints and agility drills are designed to increase your lactic acid threshold. As you advance through the program, you will be able to run faster and recover quicker between these sprints and drills. The alactic and lactic acid management systems and exercise modalities used in the Daily Workout Guide are ideal for the development of lean muscle in conjunction with your nutrition, supplementation, and strength-management programs.

To keep fatigue levels under control, the most intense parts of the workout, designed to build pure speed and reaction, are placed early on the workout days following rest and recovery days. Exercises to build leg strength are placed on alternating days early in the workout to maximize strength. Pay close attention to the sequence of the exercises and drills and do not change the format unless advised to by your physician, trainer, or health-care professional.

Flexibility exercises are an important part of each workout day because they help you to maximize your range of motion in speed-related muscle groups.

Since cardiovascular exercises are done in the presence of oxygen, which minimizes the buildup of lactic acid, I provide an *optional* cardio exercise schedule for days 3 or 6. I recommend doing at least one cardio day per week since excess cardio training is not conducive to lean muscle growth. While cardiovascular training will give you a lactic acid clearance period between high-intensity workouts, a cardio day really is optional because just performing the Lean and Hard Workouts four days a week will automatically increase your cardiovascular capacity. In fact, program participants achieved a 30 percent improvement in their cardiovascular base with very limited direct cardio activity.

Your four-day workout routine is the only mandatory exercise I am asking you to perform if you want to achieve maximum muscle-building results in only six weeks.

Day 1   Pure speed and reaction
             Upper body strength and core development

Day 2	Lower body strength and core development
	Speed endurance and leg strength
Day 3	Rest and recovery day or
	Optional cardiovascular/upper and lower core development
Day 4	Pure speed and reaction
	Upper body strength and core development
Day 5	Lower body strength and core development
	Speed endurance and leg strength
Day 6	Rest and recovery day or
	Optional cardiovascular/upper and lower core development
Day 7	Rest and recovery day

Performing High-Intensity Training

Before you begin your HIT workout, there are a few things that you should keep in mind.

Always make sure that you carefully warm up and cool down as directed before, during, and after this exercise program. As you can see in the Lean and Hard Daily Workout Guide in the next chapter, I suggest the following general warm-up: jogging 440 yards or using a stationary device such as a treadmill or a bicycle for 5 minutes at a rate of perceived exertion (RPE) of 4, then stretching out your lower body. Your speed-improvement drills comprise the next part of your warm-up. Cooldowns involve walking and jogging the designated number of yards at an RPE of 4, then stretching your upper or lower body, depending upon which part of your body you will be exercising on that particular day.

Orient yourself with the drills and the equipment. Before you begin the Lean and Hard Workout, make sure that you are familiar with each of the components. This will save you time and help you to maintain the intensity of your training. Practice the speed-improvement drills to make sure that you can perform each one correctly. Familiarize yourself with the selectorized weight training machines and dumbbell exercises that you plan to use in your gym. If you have any questions, ask one of the gym's trainers to show you how to properly position your body for each exercise and demonstrate proper lifting and breathing techniques. He or she can also help you to select the proper starting weight for each dumbbell set or machine.

Be patient with yourself if you need to keep referring to the instructions in this book during your first couple of workouts. Very soon you will become familiar with all of the routines.

When you are using a machine or dumbbells, lift only the amount of weight that you can comfortably handle, depending upon the required number of reps and sets and the body part you are working. The correct amount of weight will be enough to make you feel as if you have reached the point of muscle fatigue by the end of your required reps. If you are lifting too much weight, you won't be able to complete the set. Too little weight and you won't feel muscle tiredness at the end of your reps. Each lifting stroke should be relatively slow, with a well-controlled return. A good rule of thumb is to lift on a count of two and let down the weight on a count of four. If you are not sure how much weight you should be lifting, ask a trainer. Don't risk injuring yourself.

Advance in the program over time as you get stronger and develop an enhanced ability to recover between the exercises. Attempt to increase your weight by approximately *five pounds each week* or so to keep your body changing, but *never* compromise your form, stability, alignment, or posture to increase the number of pounds you are lifting. The result is almost certain to be injury and poor posture. The best way to build strength is to maintain proper position and form during your workout, even if you are using only a relatively light amount of weight. Play it safe and never try to handle more weight than your body can stabilize.

Remember to consistently take your high-performance nutritional supplementation. The supplements you take before, during, and after your workout help to improve your energy system's ability to tolerate the intensity of the workout and aid in recovery between training days.

Try to complete all repetitions for each machine or dumbbell routine. If the weight becomes heavy, stop the set, reduce the weight, and continue until you have completed the number of repetitions.

Maintain correct body positioning. The most efficient position for the body while doing high-intensity resistance training is one in which the spine is in a neutral position with a slight degree of straightening in the thoracic region (upper back). This is accomplished by positioning yourself comfortably against the backrest of the machine or the bench, then pushing your shoulders back slightly (known as "scapular retraction") and lifting your chest slightly up and out. Positioning the spine in this manner is more efficient for supporting weight while still allowing for the least amount of intervertebral disk compression in the cervical (neck) and lumbar (lower back) regions. Also contract your abdominal muscles during lifting to help stabilize the lumbar spine.

Don't forget to breathe—breathing will keep your blood pressure from rising. Depending on the exercise, exhale when you extend and inhale on the way back in; inhale on the way down and exhale on the way up.

Stay hydrated. When exercising, make sure that you carry a bottle of water or a bottle of your favorite multidextrin-based sports drink, such as Poweraid, mixed with glucose polymers and take frequent drinks. You will want to drink between half and one entire 1.5-liter bottle of liquid per hour of workout time.

Finish your workout with a cooldown to decrease your pulse and breathing rates, again, by walking or jogging the designated number of yards or using a stationary device for 5 minutes. Gradually reduce the intensity level until your pulse returns to a normal resting state. Then perform some easy stretching exercises to loosen tight muscles and increase flexibility.

Develop a maintenance program. Once you have completed the 6-week Lean and Hard Program, I have provided a system to enable you to maintain your muscle gains (see page 204). Keep in mind, however, that you may wish to adjust this maintenance program over time, depending upon your age and your different objectives and goals. No body or life stays the same as the years go by, so from time to time you may wish to consult a trainer regarding how you might substitute different resistance exercises while working the same muscle groups.

How to Perform the Lean and Hard Resistance Exercises

To help you work out correctly and get the most out of each set, I have included photographs and verbal descriptions of each exercise specifying your body position and how you should perform each motion.

You may already be familiar with some of these exercises. If so, I suggest that you read the descriptions anyway to check your form.

You will find a Lean and Hard Daily Workout Guide in chapter 11, which gives you a detailed description of the order and duration of each of the warm-ups, drills, buildups, and resistance exercises. This guide is set up to make each workout as efficient and easy to follow as possible.

Again, while this program has proven to be extremely safe for adults of all fitness levels, I do not advise you to attempt to build lean muscle without proper medical supervision. I strongly recommend that you work in conjunction with your doctor on the implementation of this exercise program. He or she can tell you if you have any preexisting condition or potential for any disease process that would keep you from performing high-intensity training at this time. If so, there are programs you can follow that will help you to build up to the Lean and Hard Workout (see my book *Maximum Energy for Life*).

CHEST

Dumbbell Chest Press

Positioning: Plant your feet firmly on the ground or on an elevated platform. Place your sacrum, head, and shoulder blades flat against the bench (remember to contract your shoulder blades). Keep a natural arch in your lower back. Align your arms straight up from the shoulders with your elbows rotated outward and slightly flexed.

Motion: Bend both elbows and lower arms so that your upper arms from a 90-degree angle with your sides. Without rotating your elbow or shoulder, continue down until your upper arm is parallel to the floor and forms a 90-degree angle with your forearm. Contract your chest and push your arms up to your starting position along the same path.

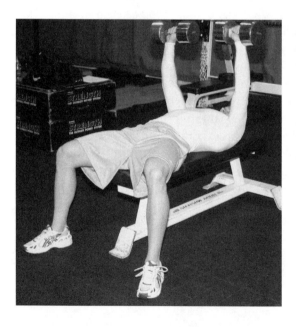
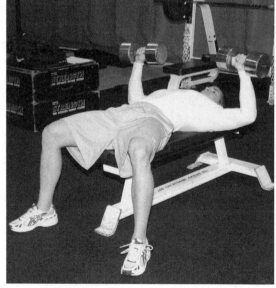

Barbell Chest Press

Positioning: Plant your feet firmly on the ground or on an elevated platform. Place your sacrum, head, and shoulder blades flat against the bench. Keep a natural arch in your lower back. Grasp the bar in such a manner as to form a 90-degree angle at the elbow when the bar is lowered. Begin by holding the bar with your arms straight from the shoulders and your elbows rotated out and slightly flexed.

Motion: Bend both elbows and lower the bar straight down so that your upper arms form a 90-degree angle with your sides. Without rotating your shoulders, continue down until your upper arms are parallel to the floor and form a 90-degree angle with your forearms. Contract your chest and push your arms up to your starting position along the same path.

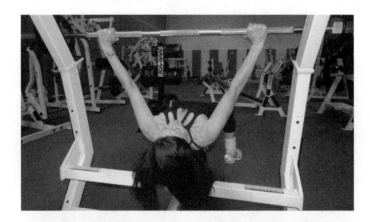

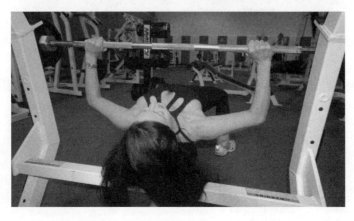

Incline Chest Press

Positioning: Plant your feet firmly on the ground or on an elevated platform. Place your sacrum, head, and shoulder blades flat against the bench inclined at about a 20-degree angle. Keep a natural arch in your lower back. Align your arms straight up from the shoulders with your elbows rotated out and slightly flexed.

Motion: Bend both elbows and lower arms so that your upper arm forms about a 90-degree angle with your sides. Without rotating your elbow or shoulder, continue until your upper arms form a 90-degree angle with your forearms. Contract your chest and push your arms up to your starting position along the same path.

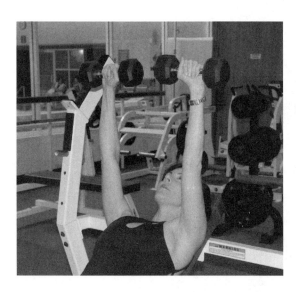
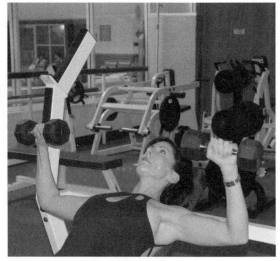

ARMS

Biceps Curl

Positioning: Stand with your feet about shoulder width apart and your knees and hips slightly flexed. Keep your upper arms firmly at your sides and hold the dumbbells with your lower arms and wrists facing forward. Align your elbows below the shoulders and flex slightly.

Motion: Contract your biceps, flex your elbows, and bring both forearms up toward the upper arms to just past 90 degrees. Do not move your upper arms throughout. Lower the dumbbells back to your starting position along the same path.

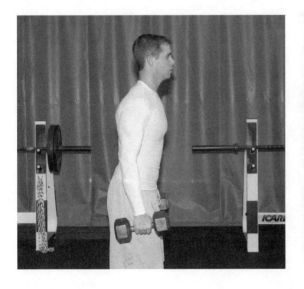
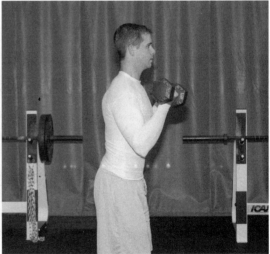

Dumbbell Triceps Extension

Positioning: Plant your feet firmly on the ground or on an elevated platform. Place your sacrum, head, and shoulder blades flat against the bench. Maintain a natural arch in your lower back. Hold your arms straight up above your shoulders with your elbows slightly flexed and pointing toward your feet.

Motion: Slowly lower your forearms down without moving your shoulders or upper arms. Continue to lower your forearms, keeping them parallel to each other and aligned with your shoulders until they form a 90-degree angle with your upper arms. Hold for a second, then return to your starting position along the same path.

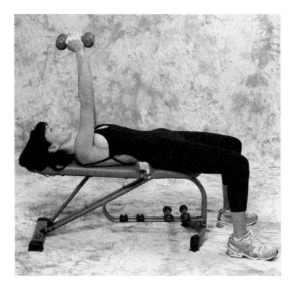
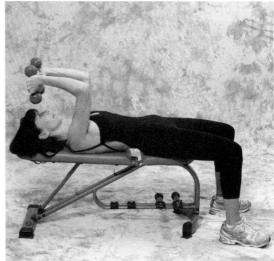

Triceps Pressdown

Positioning: Stand in front of the cable machine with your feet about shoulder width apart, knees and hips slightly bent. Hold your upper arms firmly against the sides of your body throughout. Grasp the bar overhand, placing your hands at a width that is aligned with your elbows and upper arms. Begin with your arms straight down and your elbows aligned under your shoulders, pointed back and slightly flexed.

Motion: Slowly let your forearms be pulled up and in front of your body. Continue until they form a 90-degree angle with your upper arms. Hold for a moment, then slowly pull the lower arms back down to their original position along the same path.

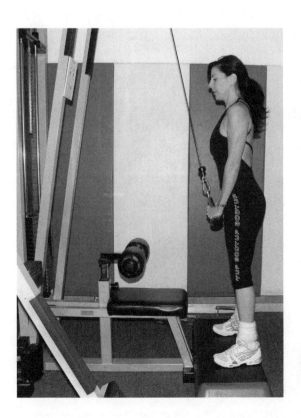 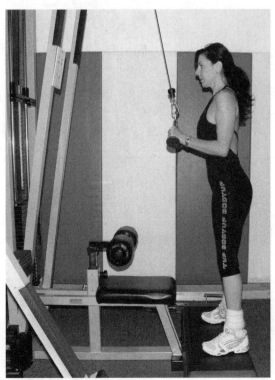

BACK

Lat Pulldown

Positioning: Place your hands on the bar so that when your upper arms are parallel to the floor, they form a 90-degree angle with your forearms. Sit with your knees under the pad and lean back until you reach a 20- to 50-degree angle. Maintain a natural arch in your lower back.

Motion: Contract your lats and pull the bar down until your upper arms are parallel to the floor. Hold for a moment, then return to your starting position along the same path.

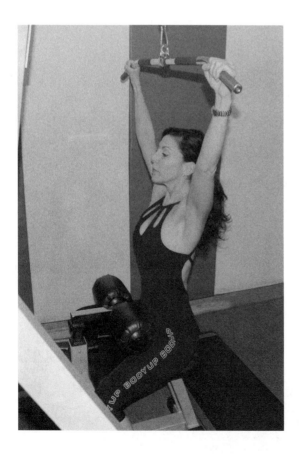
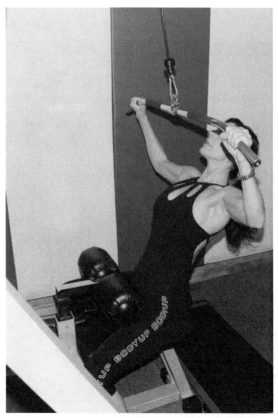

One Arm Bent-Over Row

Positioning: Place one knee on the bench at an equal height to the other knee. Flex your hips and knees and plant one hand on the bench so that your upper body is at a 60- to 90-degree angle to the floor. Hold the dumbbell straight down with your elbow slightly flexed. Flex your stationary arm slightly. Keep a natural arch in your lower back.

Motion: Pull the dumbbell straight up, keeping it close to the side of your body. Continue until your elbow is at a 90-degree angle. Hold for a moment, then slowly return to your starting position along the same path.

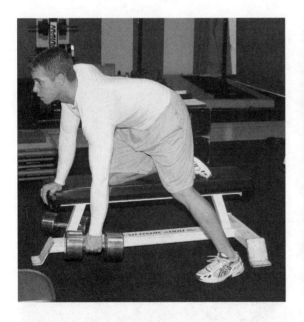
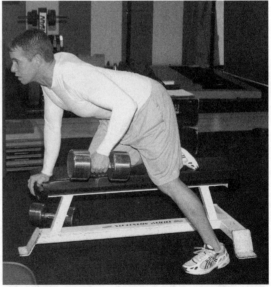

SHOULDERS

Front Deltoid Flexion

Positioning: Stand with your feet about shoulder width apart and your knees and hips slightly flexed. Hold the dumbbells parallel to your body with your wrists facing in and your elbows pointing back, slightly flexed. Begin with your arms slightly forward so that there is some resistance.

Motion: Pull your arms up and slightly out, keeping your hands relaxed and your elbows slightly flexed. Continue until your arms are parallel to the floor with your hands just slightly more than shoulder width apart. Hold for a moment, then slowly return to your starting position along the same path.

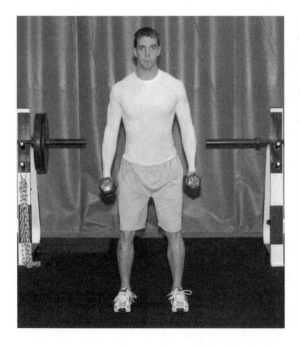
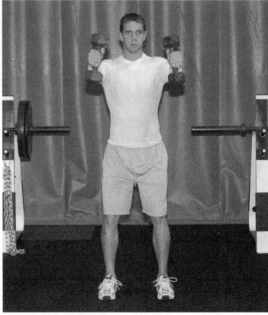

Side Deltoid Raise

Positioning: Stand with your feet about shoulder width apart and your knees and hips flexed. Lean forward slightly so that your shoulders are approximately aligned with your knees. Hold the dumbbells parallel to your body with your wrists facing in and your elbows pointing back, slightly flexed. Maintain a natural arch in your lower back. Begin with your arms slightly away from your sides so that there is some resistance.

Motion: Pull your arms up and out, keeping a slight flex in your elbows. Continue until your arms are slightly below parallel to the floor, about 80 degrees. Hold for a moment, then slowly return to your starting position along the same path.

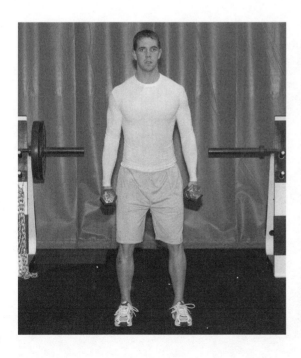 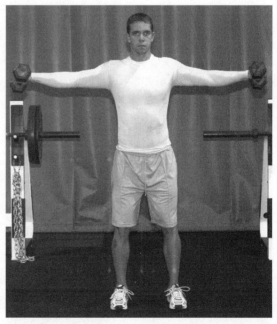

Rear Deltoid Row

Positioning: Face into an adjustable incline bench. Lean forward so that your upper body is 45 to 75 degrees to the floor. Maintain a natural arch in your lower back. Let your arms hang straight down with your wrists facing back and your elbows pointing to the side, slightly flexed.

Motion: Bending at the elbows and shoulders, pull the weight straight up until your upper arms are parallel to the floor and form a 90-degree angle with your forearms. Remember to contract your abdominal muscles to protect your back. Hold for a moment, then return to your starting position along the same path.

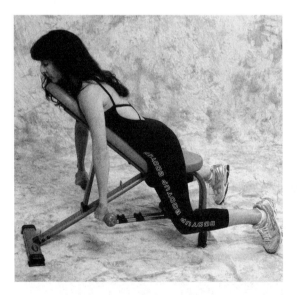
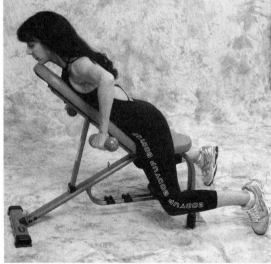

Front Shoulder Press

Positioning: Sit on the end of the bench with your feet flat on the floor. Hold the dumbbells out in front of your chest with your palms facing forward and your arms forming 90-degree angles. Keep your back straight with a natural arch in your lower back. It may be helpful to use a bench with a backrest set close to 90 degrees.

Motion: Push the dumbbells straight up as high as possible without letting them travel back beyond the center line of your body. At full extension, pause for a moment, then return to your starting position, being careful not to come down below 90 degrees.

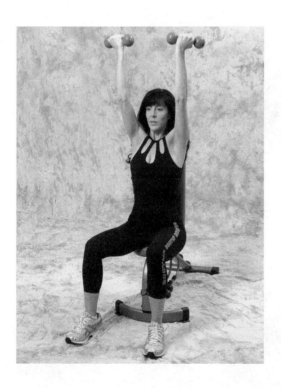
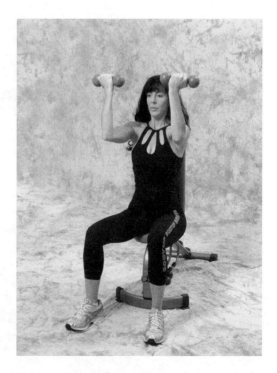

ROTATOR CUFF

Dumbbell Internal Rotation

Positioning: Lie on the floor or a mat on your side with your bottom elbow in front of your waist for support. Hold the dumbbell with your bottom hand and lay your forearm out perpendicular to your body. You may choose to place a towel or a pillow under your head to support your neck. Roll up a small towel and place it under your working armpit. Squeeze your arm against the towel to isolate the anterior shoulder muscle.

Motion: Keeping your upper arm motionless, bring the weight up to your body. Maintain a 90-degree angle between your upper and lower arm throughout. Hold for a moment, then return to your starting position along the same path.

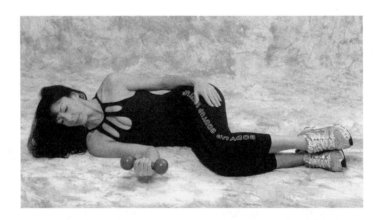

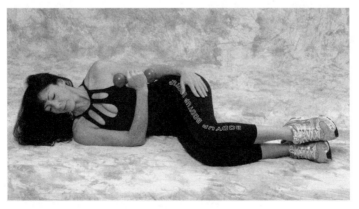

Dumbbell External Rotation

Positioning: Lie on the ground on your side with your bottom arm under your head for support. Hold a dumbbell in your upper hand. Keep your upper arm against the side of your body and let your forearm hang across your body so that the elbow is bent at a 90-degree angle. Be sure to support your neck. Place a towel under the targeted arm to help achieve proper form. Roll up a small towel and place it under your working armpit. Squeeze your arm against the towel to isolate the supraspinatus.

Motion: Raise the weight toward the ceiling until it is perpendicular to the ground. Do not rotate any farther. Keep your upper arm against the side of your body and maintain a 90-degree angle between your upper and lower arm throughout. Hold for a moment, then return to your starting position along the same path.

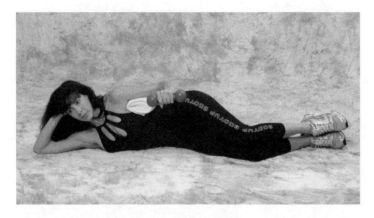

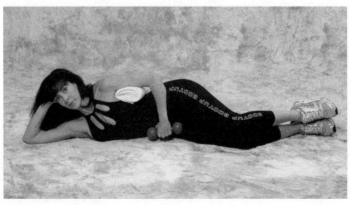

LEGS

Leg Press

Positioning: (The machine you are using may vary somewhat from the one featured in the photograph.) Lie down with your sacrum and shoulder blades pressed firmly against the back pad. Keep a natural arch in your lower back. Extend both legs straight out, aligned with your hips. Keep your feet pointed straight ahead. Begin with your legs fully extended.

Motion: Bend your knees slowly until your upper and lower leg form a 90-degree angle. Keep your heels in contact with the platform at all times. Hold for a moment and slowly extend your legs back to their starting position. Resist locking your legs and lifting your upper body off the pad throughout the motion. Do not allow your knees to extend past your toes.

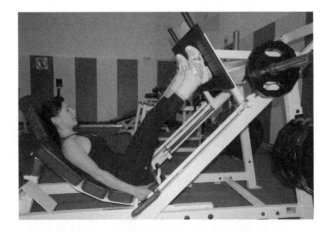

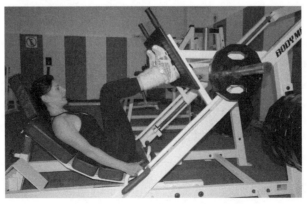

Bridge

Positioning: Lie down with your sacrum and shoulder blades flat on the floor. Bend at the knees and waist and place your feet flat on the ground so that your upper and lower leg form about a 90-degree angle. Place your hands alongside your body or cross them over your chest.

Motion: Slowly push your hips and pelvis region up while holding your feet and shoulders firmly against the ground. Continue until your upper body and thighs form a straight line. Hold for a moment and return to your starting position. Do not lift your head off the ground, which will put undue stress on your neck. For a single-leg bridge, cross one leg over the other and repeat the exercise. You may hold a light dumbbell in your hands across your lower abs for added resistance.

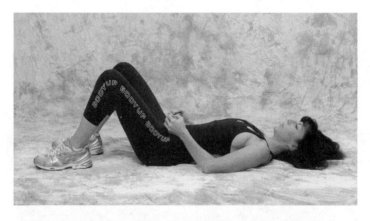

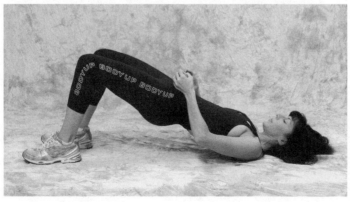

Lunge

Positioning: Stand with your legs aligned directly under your hips, your feet pointed forward, and your knees slightly flexed. Place one leg slightly in front of the other, with your hip and knee bent more and your weight on the ball of that foot. Keep your upper body straight up and down, with most of your weight on the stationary leg.

Motion: Contract your abdominal muscle to protect your back. Take a long stride forward with the lead leg, landing softly on your heel while keeping your upper body straight. Continue to lower your body until your lead leg forms a 90-degree angle. At this point your trail leg will be slightly flexed and your lower back will have a natural arch. Hold for a moment, then pull the trail leg and your body back up to your starting position and step again. Do the required number of reps while alternating legs. Do not allow the knee of the lead leg to extend past the toe during the lunge.

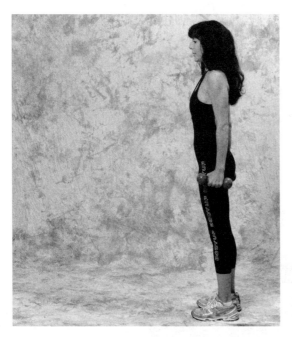
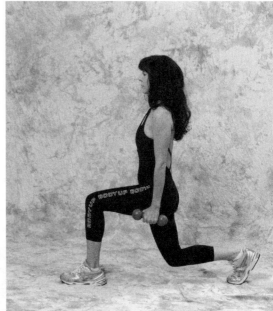

Hamstring Curl

Positioning: (The machine you are using may vary somewhat from the one featured in the photograph.) Lie on your stomach with your legs together and your knees at the end of the pad. Hold both handles firmly, turn your head to the side, and press your hips firmly against the pad. Begin with your knees flexed and the weight lifted slightly so that there is resistance.

Motion: Pull your lower legs up slowly, keeping your hips against the pad. Continue until your hamstrings are fully contracted and your knees lift off the pad slightly. Hold for a moment, then lower your legs down to your starting position. This exercise may also be done one leg at a time. Do not curl past 90 degrees.

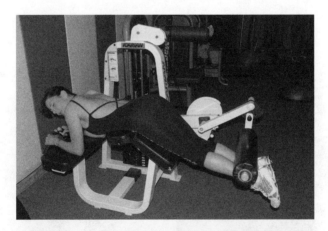

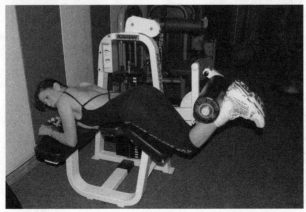

Calf Raise

Positioning: Stand with your legs and feet straight and the balls of your feet on an elevated platform. Slightly flex your knees throughout the motion. Begin with your heels below your toes and tension in your calves.

Motion: Contract your calves and pull up your heels, keeping a slight knee bend and a natural arch in your lower back. Continue until your ankles are fully extended. Hold for a moment, then slowly return to your starting position, keeping your upper body as still as possible.

You should also perform calf raises in two other positions:

1. Point your toes in and your heels out from each other to slightly alter the focus muscles.
2. Point your toes out and your heels in for another variation.

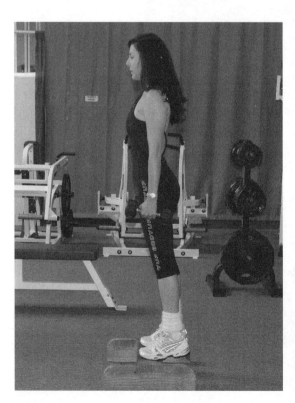
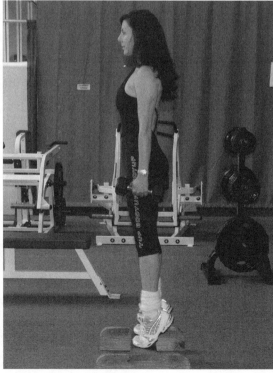

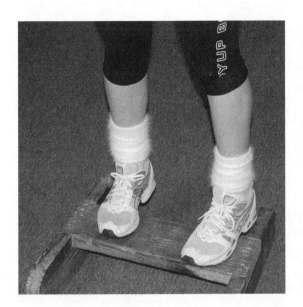

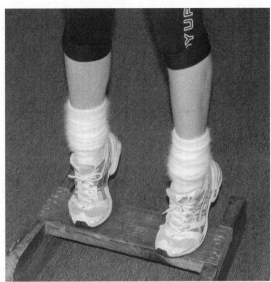

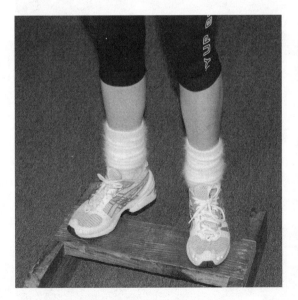

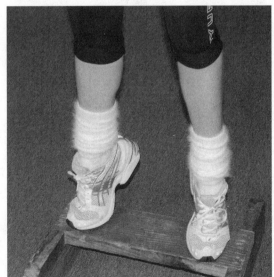

HIPS

Hip Adduction

Positioning: (The machine you are using may vary somewhat from the one featured in the photograph.) Stand facing the machine with your hips aligned with your center axis and the pad placed just above your knee. Hold the bars with your arms straight out to the side and your elbows slightly flexed. Place the leg being exercised on top of the pad below the knee and extend out 20 to 40 degrees, or as far as possible without leaning. Keep your leg straight and maintain a natural arch in your lower back.

Motion: Pull your leg down slowly while keeping it straight and a natural arch in your lower back. Continue until the heel of your active leg is directly aligned with the toe of your stationary leg, or as far forward as you can move it without losing your form or leaning. Hold for a moment, then slowly bring your leg back up to its original position. Perform the prescribed number of reps for each leg, then move to the other leg.

Hip adduction can also be performed with a cable or a flexible rubber cord. Set the cable or the cord low and repeat the above motion.

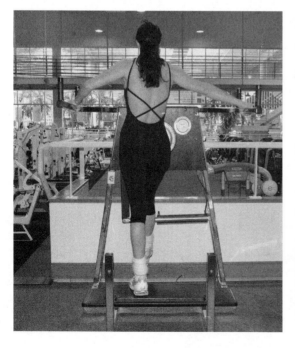
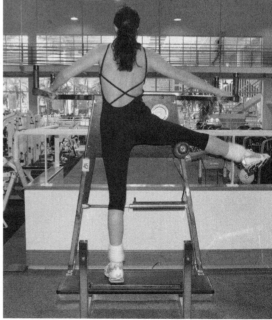

Hip Abduction

Positioning: (The machine you are using may vary somewhat from the one featured in the photograph.) Stand facing the machine with your hips aligned with your center axis and the pad just above your knee. Hold the bar with your arms straight out and your elbows slightly flexed. Begin with the pad on the outside of the knee of the leg being exercised and align your heel with the toe of the stationary leg. Maintain a natural arch in your lower back.

Motion: Pull your leg up and out slowly, keeping it as straight as possible. Continue out to 20 to 40 degrees or as far as possible without leaning or losing form. Hold for a moment, then slowly bring your leg back to your starting position. Perform the prescribed number of reps for each leg.

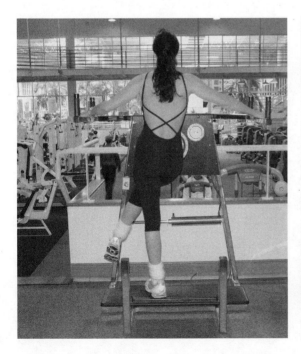
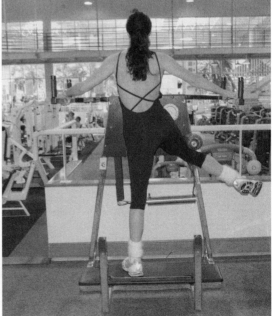

TRUNK AND ABDOMINALS

No weight is required for these exercises. To increase the intensity of the workout, increase your number of repetitions.

Be certain to properly stretch your hip flexors after performing these exercises.

Upper Trunk Flexion

Positioning: Lie on the ground or on a flat platform with your back flat and your sacrum firmly against the pad. Flex your hips and knees to form a 90-degree angle and elevate your legs on a chair, bench, or exercise ball. Rotate your hips and feet out 20 to 30 degrees. Begin with your arms crossed over your chest or placed on either side of your head at your temples. Do not place your hands behind your head or neck.

Motion: Contract your abdominals and pull your rib cage up 6 to 12 inches toward your pelvis. Continue until your abdominals are fully contracted, keeping your sacrum flat against the pad. Hold for a moment, then slowly return to your starting position. Be sure not to lift your lower back off the pad throughout. Move your chin toward your chest to help you achieve proper form. Do not raise your head and neck off the ground at an angle greater than 45 degrees (with your chin in a neutral position).

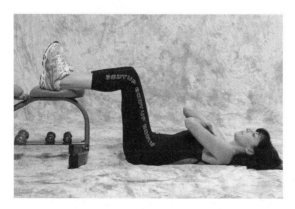 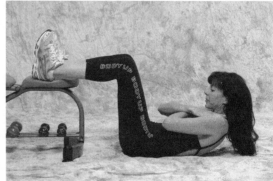

Lower Trunk Flexion

Positioning: Lie on the ground or on a flat platform with your back flat and your sacrum firmly against the pad. With your legs together, flex your hips and knees to form a 90-degree angle. Hold firmly to the back side of the platform or put the palms of your hands firmly on the stationary surface. Flatten your lower back against the pad. Begin with your hips slightly raised for tension.

Motion: Contract your abdominals and pull your pelvis up 2 to 4 inches toward your rib cage. Continue until your abdominals are fully contracted and your hips are off the pad as far as possible. Hold for a moment, then slowly return to your starting position. Be sure to keep your upper back flat against the pad throughout.

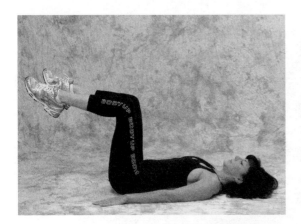
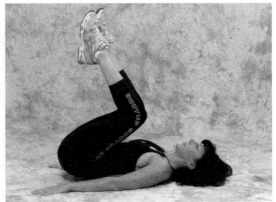
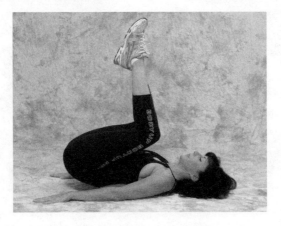

Back Raise

Positioning: Lie facedown on a flat or inclined platform. Spread your legs about shoulder width apart and place your arms alongside your body. Begin with your head and chest raised slightly off the pad with slight tension in your lower back.

Motion: Slowly raise your trunk and pull your shoulder blades back. Continue until your lower back is fully contracted or as far as possible without any spinal discomfort. Hold for a moment, then slowly lower your trunk back to your starting position. Keep your pelvis pressed firmly against the pad and avoid rotating, twisting, or rolling your trunk or legs throughout. Keep your head and neck in a relaxed, comfortable position throughout.

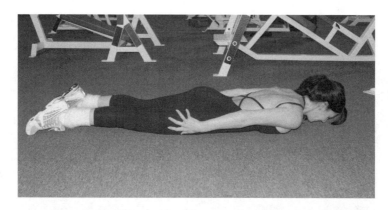

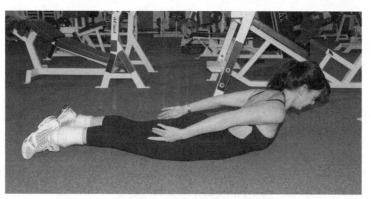

Opposite Arm and Leg Raise (Aquaman or Aquawoman)

Positioning: Lie facedown on a flat surface with both arms extended comfortably overhead and your legs straight. Rest your forehead on a towel or turn your head to one side. Begin with one arm and the opposite leg raised slightly off the ground to provide tension.

Motion: Slowly raise your arm and the opposite leg straight up, about 4 inches, keeping your head and pelvis firmly on the ground. Contract your buttocks as you lift your arm and leg. Hold for a moment, then return to your starting position. Switch your arm and leg and repeat. Avoid rotating, twisting, or rolling your body in any way throughout.

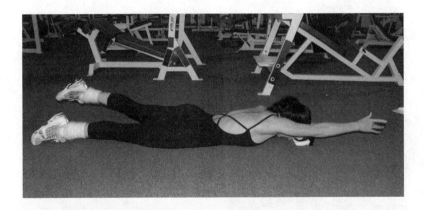

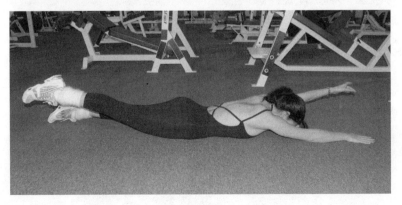

Seated Rotation

Positioning: Sit on the floor with your knees bent and your feet crossed at the ankles. You have the option of holding a light weight (dumbbell, medicine ball, or weight plate) in front of your chest with both arms extended. Tighten your abdominals and raise your feet slightly off the ground.

Motion: Twist your upper body to one side, following the weight with your head and eyes. Continue as far as possible without losing form or leaning. Hold for a moment, then return to your starting position. Repeat the motion on the other side. Throughout the motion, avoid bending over at the waist. Keep your upper body straight up with the appropriate lean, and keep your feet several inches off the ground. Contract your abs during the exercise.

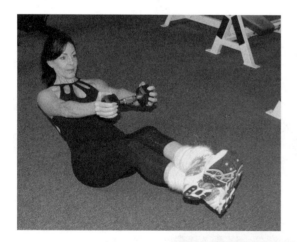 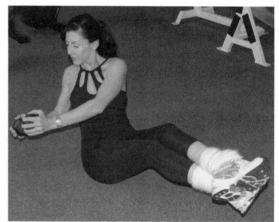

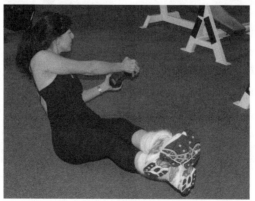

Andrea: The Best Shape of My Life

Andrea was one of the people who accepted the challenge to be part of the original Lean and Hard Study at Louisiana State University Health Care Network. She got back in touch with me recently because she wanted to do another six weeks on the workout. She told me that recently she had found a photograph of herself standing next to a trail bike at Canyon Ranch a short time after she'd finished the program. "I couldn't believe how fantastic I looked. I was in the absolute best shape of my life. I want to get there again."

Andrea reminisced about an evening when she and I had attended a New Orleans fund-raiser. We were talking to group of people about the Lean and Hard Workout and one listener was scoffing. "He gave Mackie—a lean, toned 5' 9" man who was then in his late forties—a dare: 'I'll bet you can't do fifty push-ups.'

"I chimed in and said, 'I trained in Mackie's program and I can do twenty men's push-ups. I can do thirty.'

'There's no way you can do thirty men's push-ups!' the guy said."

To everyone's surprise, Andrea dropped to the floor in her evening gown and white gloves and did thirty push-ups. "No one could believe it," she recalled. "My muscles were incredible. There's a picture that someone took of me that night. You can see my toned arms. There's this bravado that goes with that look that energizes you.

"Being fit is contagious. It's self-motivating. Once you're in that zone, the high you get is your motivation to continue with the plan. For me all I needed to help me get into that zone was having a set schedule, a set routine."

Andrea originally took the Lean and Hard Workout challenge because she was tired of never being able to drop that last six or seven pounds. Once she got started she was shocked at how fast her body changed. "I was surprised how quickly people began taking notice of me in a matter of only a few weeks, especially the people in the gym who saw me with my street clothes off. They would say, "Wow! You look really great." That's motivating, when people start noticing. When you feel how strong you are and how energized you are."

Andrea is just one example of someone who got the physique she'd always wanted—and more—from the high-performance Lean and Hard Workout. Follow this program for four days a week for six weeks and you'll be amazed at the results.

11

The Lean and Hard Workout

When I asked one of the women who had completed the Lean and Hard Program what she liked best about the workout, she said, "A lot of people feel like they need a trainer, and I used to think I was one of them. But I live in a city where trainers are fifty or sixty dollars an hour, and I can't really afford that. That's what ignited me to get on this program, because I needed something I could do on my own.

"And this worked for me. It really gave me a sense of discipline because everything was spelled out exactly. It was easy to follow, like a trainer in a book. It's a great way to get to your target goal."

When I designed this program, that was precisely my goal, to give you clear and specific instructions to get the most muscle-building potential out of each high-intensity training session. Below you will find your daily schedule of exercises for your HIT workout. Remember to perform all of the exercises in the order shown. Make sure that you complete all sets and reps of *every exercise in each individual segment* before moving on to the next segment.

As with the performance nutrition supplementation schedule, always remember that *timing* is an important factor in determining how much you will get out of your Lean and Hard HIT Workout. A recent article published in *Medicine and Science in Sports and Exercise* showed that taking no more than a one-minute rest between exercises and no more than a two- to three-minute rest between sets of high-intensity exercises "considerably elevated GH (human growth hormone) and TES (testosterone) concentrations." Remember, these are two important anabolic (muscle-building) hormones.

Again, please keep in mind that if you want something to do on your days between HIT sessions, I have provided an *optional* cardiovascular workout for days 3 or 6. However, the results you can expect from this program are not dependent upon your performing cardio. Your cardiovascular capacity will increase automatically if you simply perform the four weekly HIT workouts.

Good luck and enjoy your Lean and Hard Training Sessions!

The Lean and Hard Daily Workout Guide

Week 1, Day 1

General Warm-Up	Jog 440 yards or spend 5 minutes on a stationary device, RPE 4
	Stretch lower body
Specific Warm-Up	Skip, hip, carioca, butt kicks, backward run
SIDs, RPE 5	1 set each, 20 yards; walk back after each
	Quick feet, 10 yards, 2 sets; walk back after each
	Skip, hip, strides, 1 power transition, 30 yards
Buildups, RPE 6	2 sets, 120 yards (40-40-40)
Energy System	2 × 100 yards at 7 RPE; walk back after each
Management (Sprints)	2 × 60 yards at 8 RPE; walk back after each
	2 × 40 yards at 8 RPE; walk back after each
	Use recovery heart rate of approximately 120 bpm
Cooldown	2 × walk 50 yards, jog 50 yards, RPE 4
	Stretch upper body
Chest and Back	
Barbell chest press	4 sets, 10–12 reps, wt. _____
One arm bent-over row	4 sets, 10–12 reps, wt. _____
Shoulders	
Front shoulder flexion	3 sets, 12–15 reps, wt. _____
Side deltoid raise	3 sets, 12–15 reps, wt. _____
Rear deltoid row	3 sets, 15–20 reps, wt. _____

Rotator Cuff

    Internal rotation   2 sets, 15–20 reps, wt. _____

    External rotation   2 sets, 15–20 reps, wt. _____

Arms

    Biceps curl   3 sets, 10–12 reps, wt. _____

    Triceps pressdown   3 sets, 10–12 reps, wt. _____

Pelvic Stabilizers

    Upper trunk flexion   2 sets, 15 reps

    Seated rotation   2 sets, 10 reps

    Back raise   2 sets, 10 reps

Week 1, Day 2

General Warm-Up   Jog 440 yards or spend 5 minutes on a stationary device, RPE 4

                               Stretch lower body

Pelvic Stabilizers

    Lower trunk flexion   2 sets, 15 reps

    Seated rotation   2 sets, 10 reps

    Aquaman   2 sets, 10 reps

Hips

    Hip adduction   2 sets, 12–15 reps, wt. _____

    Hip abduction   2 sets, 12–15 reps, wt. _____

Legs

    Leg press   3 sets, 10–12 reps, wt. _____

    Hamstring curl   3 sets, 10–12 reps, wt. _____

    Walking lunge   2 sets, 10–12 reps, wt. _____

    Bridge, double leg   2 sets, 10–12 reps, wt. _____

    Calf raise   1 set, 10 reps; 1 set for each of 3 positions

General Warm-Up   Jog 440 yards or spend 5 minutes on a stationary device, RPE 4

                               Stretch lower body

Specific Warm-Up	Skip, hip, carioca, butt kicks, backward run
SIDs, RPE 5	1 set each, 20 yards; walk back after each
	Quick feet, 10 yards, 2 sets; walk back after each
	Skip, hip, strides, 1 power transition, 30 yards
Energy System	2 × 220 yards at 70–80% HR; walk back after each
Management (Sprints)	Rest at least 2 minutes
	2 × 100 yards at 70–80% HR; walk back after each
	Use recovery heart rate of approximately 130 bpm
Cooldown	2 × walk 50 yards, jog 50 yards, RPE 4
	Stretch upper body

Week 1, Day 3

Optional Cardio Day

General Warm-Up	Jog 440 yards or spend 5 minutes on a stationary device, RPE 4
	Stretch lower body
Specific Warm-Up	Stretch upper body
Pelvic Stabilizers	
Upper trunk flexion	2 sets, 15 reps
Seated rotation	2 sets, 10 reps
Back raise	2 sets, 10 reps
Cardiovascular Stationary	12 minutes on bike, stepper, or other device
Device	Stretch hip flexors
Cooldown	2 × walk 50 yards, jog 50 yards, RPE 4
	Stretch lower body
Pelvic Stabilizers	
Lower trunk flexion	2 sets, 15 reps
Seated rotation	2 sets, 10 reps
Aquaman	2 sets, 10 reps

Week 1, Day 4

General Warm-Up	Jog 440 yards or spend 5 minutes on a stationary device, RPE 4
	Stretch lower body
Specific Warm-Up	Skip, hip, carioca, butt kicks, backward run
SIDs, RPE 5	1 set each, 20 yards; walk back after each
	Quick feet, 10 yards, 2 sets; walk back after each
	Skip, hip, strides, 1 power transition, 30 yards
Buildups, RPE 6	2 sets, 120 yards (40-40-40)
Energy System	2 × 60 yards at 7 RPE; walk back after each
Management (Sprints)	2 × 40 yards at 8 RPE; walk back after each
	2 × 20 yards at 8 RPE; walk back after each
	Use recovery heart rate of approximately 120 bpm
Cooldown	2 × walk 50 yards, jog 50 yards, RPE 4
	Stretch upper body

Chest and Back

Incline chest press	4 sets, 10–12 reps, wt. _____
Lat pulldown	4 sets, 10–12 reps, wt. _____

Shoulders

Front shoulder flexion	3 sets, 12–15 reps, wt. _____
Side deltoid raise	3 sets, 12–15 reps, wt. _____
Rear deltoid row	3 sets, 15–20 reps, wt. _____

Rotator Cuff

Internal rotation	2 sets, 15–20 reps, dumbbell/cable wt. _____
External rotation	2 sets, 15–20 reps, dumbbell/cable wt. _____

Arms

Biceps curl	3 sets, 10–12 reps, wt. _____
Dumbell triceps extension	3 sets, 10–12 reps, wt. _____

Pelvic Stabilizers

Upper trunk flexion	2 sets, 15 reps
Seated rotation	2 sets, 10 reps
Back raise	2 sets, 10 reps

Week 1, Day 5

General Warm-Up

Jog 440 yards or spend 5 minutes on a stationary device, RPE 4

Stretch lower body

Pelvic Stabilizers

Lower trunk flexion	2 sets, 15–20 reps
Seated rotation	2 sets, 10 reps
Aquaman	2 sets, 15–20 reps

Hips

Hip adduction	2 sets, 12–15 reps, wt. _____
Hip abduction	2 sets, 12–15 reps, wt. _____

Legs

Leg press	3 sets, 10–12 reps, wt. _____
Hamstring curl	3 sets, 10–12 reps, wt. _____
Walking lunge	2 sets, 10–12 reps, wt. _____
Bridge, double leg	2 sets, 10–12 reps, wt. _____
Calf raise	1 set, 10 reps; 1 set for each of 3 positions

General Warm-Up

Jog 440 yards or spend 5 minutes on a stationary device, RPE 4

Stretch lower body

Specific Warm-Up

Jump rope at rookie level

Energy System Management (Shuttles)

2 × 60 yards shuttle at 70–80% HR

Rest 2 minutes between each

Use recovery heart rate of approximately 130 bpm

Cooldown	2 × walk 50 yards, jog 50 yards, RPE 4
	Stretch as needed

Week 1, Day 6

Optional cardio day; same routine as Day 3

Week 2, Day 1

General Warm-Up	Jog 440 yards or spend 5 minutes on a stationary device, RPE 4
	Stretch lower body
Specific Warm-Up	Skip, hip, carioca, butt kicks, backward run
SIDs, RPE 5	1 set each, 20 yards; walk back after each
	Quick feet, 10 yards, 2 sets; walk back after each
	Skip, hip, strides, 1 power transition, 30 yards
Buildups, RPE 6	2 sets, 120 yards (40-40-40)
Energy System	3 × 100 yards at 7 RPE; walk back after each
Management (Sprints)	3 × 60 yards at 8 RPE; walk back after each
	3 × 40 yards at 8 RPE; walk back after each
	Use recovery heart rate of approximately 120 bpm
Cooldown	2 × walk 50 yards, jog 50 yards, RPE 4
	Stretch upper body
Chest and Back	
Barbell chest press	4 sets, 10–12 reps, wt. _____
One arm bent-over row	4 sets, 10–12 reps, wt. _____
Shoulders	
Front shoulder flexion	3 sets, 12–15 reps, wt. _____
Side deltoid raise	3 sets, 12–15 reps, wt. _____
Rear deltoid row	3 sets, 15–20 reps, wt._____

Rotator Cuff

Internal rotation	2 sets, 15–20 reps, wt. _____
External rotation	2 sets, 15–20 reps, wt. _____

Arms

Biceps curl	3 sets, 10–12 reps, wt. _____
Triceps pressdown	3 sets, 10–12 reps, wt. _____

Pelvic Stabilizers

Upper trunk flexion	2 sets, 15 reps
Seated rotation	2 sets, 10 reps
Back raise	2 sets, 10 reps

Week 2, Day 2

General Warm-Up	Jog 440 yards or spend 5 minutes on a stationary device, RPE 4 Stretch lower body

Pelvic Stabilizers

Lower trunk flexion	2 sets, 15–20 reps
Seated rotation	2 sets, 10 reps
Aquaman	2 sets, 15–20 reps

Hips

Hip adduction	2 sets, 12–15 reps, wt. _____
Hip abduction	2 sets, 12–15 reps, wt. _____

Legs

Leg press	3 sets, 10–12 reps, wt. _____
Hamstring curl	3 sets, 10–12 reps, wt. _____
Walking lunge	2 sets, 10–12 reps, wt. _____
Bridge, double leg	2 sets, 10–12 reps, wt. _____
Calf raise	1 set, 10 reps; 1 set for each of 3 positions

General Warm-Up	Jog 440 yards or spend 5 minutes on a stationary device, RPE 4 Stretch lower body

Specific Warm-Up	Skip, hip, carioca, butt kicks, backward run
SIDs, RPE 5	1 set each, 20 yards; walk back after each
	Quick feet, 10 yards, 2 sets; walk back after each
	Skip, hip, strides, 1 power transition, 30 yards

Energy System	3×220 yards at 70-80% HR; walk back after each
Management (Sprints)	Rest at least 3 minutes
	3×100 yards at 70-80% HR; walk back after each
	Use recovery heart rate of approximately 130 bpm

Cooldown	$2 \times$ walk 50 yards, jog 50 yards, RPE 40%
	Stretch as needed

Week 2, Day 3

Optional Cardio Day

General Warm-Up	Jog 440 yards or spend 5 minutes on a stationary device, RPE 4
	Stretch lower body

Specific Warm-Up	Stretch upper body

Pelvic Stabilizers	
Upper trunk flexion	2 sets, 15 reps
Seated rotation	2 sets, 10 reps
Back raise	2 sets, 10 reps

Cardiovascular Stationary	15 minutes on bike, stepper, or other device
Device	Stretch hip flexors

Cooldown	$2 \times$ walk 50 yards, jog 50 yards, RPE 4
	Stretch lower body

Pelvic Stabilizers	
Lower trunk flexion	2 sets, 15–20 reps
Seated rotation	2 sets, 10 reps
Aquaman	2 sets, 15–20 reps

Week 2, Day 4

General Warm-Up	Jog 440 yards or spend 5 minutes on a stationary device, RPE 4
	Stretch lower body
Specific Warm-Up	Skip, hip, carioca, butt kicks, backward run
SIDs, RPE 5	1 set each, 20 yards; walk back after each
	Quick feet, 10 yards, 2 sets; walk back after each
	Skip, hip, strides, 1 power transition, 30 yards
Buildups, RPE 6	2 sets, 120 yards (40-40-40)
Energy System	3×60 yards at 7 RPE; walk back after each
Management (Sprints)	3×40 yards at 8 RPE; walk back after each
	3×20 yards at 8 RPE; walk back after each
	Use recovery heart rate of approximately 120 bpm
Cooldown	$2 \times$ walk 50 yards, jog 50 yards, RPE 4
	Stretch upper body

Chest and Back

Incline chest press	4 sets, 10–12 reps, wt. _____
Lat pulldown	4 sets, 10–12 reps, wt. _____

Shoulders

Front shoulder flexion	3 sets, 12–15 reps, wt. _____
Side deltoid raise	3 sets, 12–15 reps, wt. _____
Rear deltoid row	3 sets, 12–20 reps, wt. _____

Rotator Cuff

Internal rotation	2 sets, 15–20 reps, dumbbell/cable wt. _____
External rotation	2 sets, 15–20 reps, dumbbell/cable wt. _____

Arms

Alternating biceps curl	3 sets, 10–12 reps, wt. _____
Dumbbell triceps extension	3 sets, 10–12 reps, wt. _____

Pelvic Stabilizers

Upper trunk flexion	2 sets, 15 reps
Seated rotation	2 sets, 10 reps
Back raise	2 sets, 10 reps

Week 2, Day 5

General Warm-Up

Jog 440 yards or spend 5 minutes on a stationary device, RPE 4

Stretch lower body

Pelvic Stabilizers

Lower trunk flexion	2 sets, 15–20 reps
Seated rotation	2 sets, 10 reps
Aquaman	2 sets, 15–20 reps

Hips

Hip adduction	2 sets, 12–15 reps, wt. _____
Hip abduction	2 sets, 12–15 reps, wt. _____

Legs

Leg press	3 sets, 10–12 reps, wt. _____
Hamstring curl	3 sets, 10–12 reps, wt. _____
Walking lunge	2 sets, 10–12 reps, wt. _____
Bridge, double leg	2 sets, 10–12 reps, wt. _____
Calf raise	1 set, 10 reps; 1 set for each of 3 positions

General Warm-Up

Jog 440 yards or spend 5 minutes on a stationary device, RPE 4

Stretch lower body

Specific Warm-Up

Jump rope at rookie level

**Energy System
Management (Shuttles)**

3×60 yards shuttle at 70–80% max HR

Rest 2 minutes between each

Use recovery heart rate of approximately 130 bpm

Cooldown

$2 \times$ walk 50 yards, jog 50 yards, RPE 4

Stretch as needed

Week 2, Day 6

Optional cardio day; same routine as Day 3

Week 3, Day 1

General Warm-Up	Jog 440 yards or spend 5 minutes on a stationary device, RPE 4
	Stretch lower body
Specific Warm-Up	Skip, hip, carioca, butt kicks, backward run
SIDs, RPE 5	1 set each, 20 yards; walk back after each
	Quick feet, 10 yards, 2 sets; walk back after each
	Skip, hip, strides, 1 power transition, 30 yards
Buildups, RPE 6	2 sets, 120 yards (40-40-40)
Energy System	4 × 100 yards at 7 RPE; walk back after each
Management (Sprints)	4 × 60 yards at 8 RPE; walk back after each
	4 × 40 yards at 8 RPE; walk back after each
	Use recovery heart rate of approximately 120 bpm
Cooldown	2 × walk 50 yards, jog 50 yards, RPE 4
	Stretch upper body
Chest and Back	
Barbell chest press	4 sets, 8–10 reps, wt. _____
One arm bent-over row	4 sets, 8–10 reps, wt. _____
Shoulders	
Front shoulder flexion	3 sets, 10–12 reps, wt. _____
Side deltoid raise	3 sets, 10–12 reps, wt. _____
Rear deltoid row	3 sets, 10–15 reps, wt. _____
Rotator Cuff	
Internal rotation	2 sets, 20–25 reps, dumbbell/cable wt. _____
External rotation	2 sets, 20–25 reps, dumbbell/cable wt. _____

Arms

Biceps curl	3 sets, 8–10 reps, wt. _____
Triceps pressdown	3 sets, 8–10 reps, wt. _____

Pelvic Stabilizers

Upper trunk flexion	2 sets, 20 reps
Seated rotation	2 sets, 15 reps
Back raise	2 sets, 15 reps

Week 3, Day 2

General Warm-Up   Jog 440 yards or spend 5 minutes on a stationary device, RPE 4
Stretch lower body

Pelvic Stabilizers

Lower trunk flexion	2 sets, 20–25 reps
Seated rotation	2 sets, 15 reps
Aquaman	2 sets, 20–25 reps

Hips

Hip adduction	2 sets, 10–12 reps, wt. _____
Hip abduction	2 sets, 10–12 reps, wt. _____

Legs

Leg press	3 sets, 8–10 reps, wt. _____
Hamstring curl	3 sets, 8–10 reps, wt. _____
Walking lunge	2 sets, 12–15 reps, wt. _____
Bridge, double leg	2 sets, 12–15 reps, wt. _____
Calf raise	1 set to fatigue; 1 set for each of 3 positions

General Warm-Up   Jog 440 yards or spend 5 minutes on a stationary device, RPE 4
Stretch lower body

Specific Warm-Up   Skip, hip, carioca, butt kicks, backward run
SIDs, RPE 5   1 set each, 20 yards; walk back after each
Quick feet, 10 yards, 2 sets; walk back after each
Skip, hip, strides, 1 power transition, 30 yards

Energy System Management (Sprint)	4 × 220 yards at 70–80% HR; walk back after each
	Rest at least 4 minutes
	4 × 100 yards at 70–80% HR; walk back after each
	Use recovery heart rate of approximately 130 bpm
Cooldown	2 × walk 50 yards, jog 50 yards, RPE 4
	Stretch as needed

Week 3, Day 3

Optional Cardio Day

General Warm-Up	Jog 440 yards or spend 5 minutes on a stationary device, RPE 4
	Stretch lower body
Specific Warm-Up	Stretch upper body
Pelvic Stabilizers	
Upper trunk flexion	2 sets, 20 reps
Seated rotation	2 sets, 15 reps
Back raise	2 sets, 15 reps
Cardiovascular Stationary Device	17 minutes on bike, stepper, or other device
	Stretch hip flexors
Cooldown	2 × walk 50 yards, jog 50 yards, RPE 4
	Stretch lower body
Pelvic Stabilizers	
Lower trunk flexion	2 sets, 20–25 reps
Seated rotation	2 sets, 15 reps
Aquaman	2 sets, 20–25 reps

Week 3, Day 4

General Warm-Up	Jog 440 yards or spend 5 minutes on a stationary device, RPE 4
	Stretch lower body

Specific Warm-Up	Skip, hip, carioca, butt kicks, backward run
SIDs, RPE 5	1 set each, 20 yards; walk back after each
	Quick feet, 10 yards, 2 sets; walk back after each
	Skip, hip, strides, 1 power transition, 30 yards
Buildups, RPE 6	2 sets, 120 yards (40-40-40)
Energy System	3 × 60 yards at 7 RPE; walk back after each
Management (Sprints)	3 × 40 yards at 8 RPE; walk back after each
	3 × 20 yards at 8 RPE; walk back after each
	Use recovery heart rate of approximately 120 bpm
Cooldown	2 × walk 50 yards, jog 50 yards, RPE 4
	Stretch upper body

Chest and Back

Incline chest press	4 sets, 10–12 reps, wt. _____
Lat pulldown	4 sets, 10–12 reps, wt. _____

Shoulders

Front shoulder flexion	3 sets, 12–15 reps, wt. _____
Side deltoid raise	3 sets, 12–15 reps, wt. _____
Rear deltoid row	3 sets, 15–20 reps, wt. _____

Rotator Cuff

Internal rotation	2 sets, 15–20 reps, wt. _____
External rotation	2 sets, 15–20 reps, wt. _____

Arms

Alternating biceps curl	3 sets, 10–12 reps, wt. _____
Dumbbell triceps extension	3 sets, 10–12 reps, wt. _____

Pelvic Stabilizers

Upper trunk flexion	2 sets, 15 reps
Seated rotation	2 sets, 10 reps
Back raise	2 sets, 10 reps

Week 3, Day 5

General Warm-Up	Jog 440 yards or spend 5 minutes on a stationary device, RPE 4
	Stretch lower body

Pelvic Stabilizers

Lower trunk flexion	2 sets, 20–25 reps
Seated rotation	2 sets, 15 reps
Aquaman	2 sets, 20–25 reps

Hips

Hip adduction	2 sets, 10–12 reps, wt. _____
Hip abduction	2 sets, 10–12 reps, wt. _____

Legs

Leg press	3 sets, 8–10 reps, wt. _____
Hamstring curl	3 sets, 8–10 reps, wt. _____
Walking lunge	2 sets, 12–15 reps, wt. _____
Bridge, double leg	2 sets, 12–15 reps, wt. _____
Calf raise	1 set to fatigue; 1 set for each of 3 positions

General Warm-Up	Jog 440 yards or spend 5 minutes on a stationary device, RPE 4
	Stretch lower body
Specific Warm-Up	Jump rope at minor league level
Energy System Management (Shuttles)	1 × 100 yards shuttle at 70–80% HR
	1 × 60 yards shuttle at 70–80% HR
	Rest 2 minutes between each
	Use recovery heart rate of approximately 130 bpm
Cooldown	2 × walk 50 yards, jog 50 yards, RPE 4
	Stretch as needed

Week 3, Day 6

Optional cardio day; same routine as Day 3

Week 4, Day 1

General Warm-Up	Jog 440 yards or spend 5 minutes on a stationary device, RPE 4
	Stretch lower body
Specific Warm-Up	Skip, hip, carioca, butt kicks, backward run
SIDs, RPE 5	1 set each, 20 yards; walk back after each
	Quick feet, 10 yards, 2 sets; walk back after each
	Skip, hip, strides, 1 power transition, 30 yards
Buildups, RPE 6	2 sets, 120 yards (40-40-40)
Energy System	2×100 yards at 7 RPE; walk back after each
Management (Sprints)	3×60 yards at 8 RPE; walk back after each
	3×40 yards at 8 RPE; walk back after each
	3×20 yards at near max; walk back after each
	Use recovery heart rate of approximately 120 bpm
Cooldown	$2 \times$ walk 50 yards, jog 50 yards, RPE 4
	Stretch upper body

Chest and Back

Barbell chest press	4 sets, 8–10 reps, wt. _____
One arm bent-over row	4 sets, 8–10 reps, wt. _____

Shoulders

Front shoulder flexion	3 sets, 10–12 reps, wt. _____
Side deltoid raise	3 sets, 10–12 reps, wt. _____
Rear deltoid row	3 sets, 12–15 reps, wt. _____

Rotator Cuff

Internal rotation	2 sets, 20–25 reps, wt. _____
External rotation	2 sets, 20–25 reps, wt. _____

Arms

Biceps curl	3 sets, 8–10 reps, wt. _____
Triceps pressdown	3 sets, 8–10 reps, wt. _____

Pelvic Stabilizers

Upper trunk flexion	2 sets, 20 reps
Seated rotation	2 sets, 15 reps
Back raise	2 sets, 15 reps

Week 4, Day 2

General Warm-Up

Jog 440 yards or spend 5 minutes on a stationary device, RPE 4
Stretch lower body

Pelvic Stabilizers

Lower trunk flexion	2 sets, 20–25 reps
Seated rotation	2 sets, 15 reps
Aquaman	2 sets, 20–25 reps

Hips

Hip adduction	2 sets, 10–12 reps, wt. _____
Hip abduction	2 sets, 10–12 reps, wt. _____

Legs

Leg press	3 sets, 8–10 reps, wt. _____
Hamstring curl	3 sets, 8–10 reps, wt. _____
Walking lunge	2 sets, 12–15 reps, wt. _____
Bridge, double leg	2 sets, 12–15 reps, wt. _____
Calf raise	1 set to fatigue; 1 set for each of 3 positions

General Warm-Up

Jog 440 yards or spend 5 minutes on a stationary device, RPE 4
Stretch lower body

Specific Warm-Up
SIDs, RPE 5

Skip, hip, carioca, butt kicks, backward run
1 set each, 20 yards; walk back after each
Quick feet, 10 yards, 2 sets; walk back after each
Skip, hip, strides, 1 power transition, 30 yards

Energy System Management (Sprints)	4 × 220 yards at 70–80% HR; walk back after each
	Rest at least 4 minutes
	4 × 150 yards at 70–80% HR; walk back after each
	Use recovery heart rate of approximately 130 bpm
Cooldown	2 × walk 50 yards, jog 50 yards, RPE 4
	Stretch as needed

Week 4, Day 3

Optional Cardio Day

General Warm-Up	Jog 440 yards or spend 5 minutes on a stationary device, RPE 4
	Stretch lower body
Specific Warm-Up	Stretch upper body
Pelvic Stabilizers	
Upper trunk flexion	2 sets, 20 reps
Seated rotation	2 sets, 15 reps
Back raise	2 sets, 15 reps
Cardiovascular Stationary Device	19 minutes on bike, stepper, or other device
	Stretch hip flexors
Cooldown	2 × walk 50 yards, jog 50 yards, RPE 4
	Stretch lower body
Pelvic Stabilizers	
Lower trunk flexion	2 sets, 20–25 reps
Seated rotation	2 sets, 15 reps
Aquaman	2 sets, 20–25 reps

Week 4, Day 4

General Warm-Up	Jog 440 yards or spend 5 minutes on a stationary device, RPE 4
	Stretch lower body
Specific Warm-Up	Skip, hip, carioca, butt kicks, backward run
SIDs, RPE 5	1 set each, 20 yards; walk back after each
	Quick feet, 10 yards, 2 sets; walk back after each
	Skip, hip, strides, 1 power transition, 30 yards
Buildups, RPE 6	2 sets, 120 yards (40-40-40)
Energy System	2 × 60 yards at 7 RPE; walk back after each
Management (Sprints)	3 × 40 yards at 8 RPE; walk back after each
	3 × 20 yards at 8 RPE; walk back after each
	3 × 10 yards at near max; walk back after each
	Use recovery heart rate of approximately 120 bpm
Cooldown	2 × walk 50 yards, jog 50 yards, RPE 4
	Stretch upper body

Chest and Back

Incline chest press	4 sets, 8–10 reps, wt. _____
Lat pulldown	4 sets, 8–10 reps, wt. _____

Shoulders

Front shoulder flexion	3 sets, 10–12 reps, wt. _____
Side deltoid raise	3 sets, 10–12 reps, wt. _____
Rear deltoid row	3 sets, 12–15 reps, wt. _____

Rotator Cuff

Internal rotation	2 sets, 15–20 reps, wt. _____
External rotation	2 sets, 15–20 reps, wt. _____

Arms

Alternating biceps curl	3 sets, 8–10 reps, wt. _____
Dumbbell triceps extension	3 sets, 8–10 reps, wt. _____

Pelvic Stabilizers

Upper trunk flexion	2 sets, 20 reps
Seated rotation	2 sets, 15 reps
Back raise	2 sets, 15 reps

Week 4, Day 5

General Warm-Up

Jog 440 yards or spend 5 minutes on a stationary device, RPE 4
Stretch lower body

Pelvic Stabilizers

Lower trunk flexion	2 sets, 20–25 reps
Seated rotation	2 sets, 15 reps
Aquaman	2 sets, 20–25 reps

Hips

Hip adduction	2 sets, 8–10 reps, wt. _____
Hip abduction	2 sets, 8–10 reps, wt. _____

Legs

Leg press	3 sets, 8–10 reps, wt. _____
Hamstring curl	3 sets, 8–10 reps, wt. _____
Walking lunge	2 sets, 12–15 reps, wt. _____
Bridge, double leg	2 sets, 12–15 reps, wt. _____
Calf raise	1 set to fatigue; 1 set for each of 3 positions

General Warm-Up

Jog 440 yards or spend 5 minutes on a stationary device, RPE 4
Stretch lower body

Specific Warm-Up

Jump rope at minor league level

Energy System Management (Shuttles)

2 × 100 yards shuttle at 70–80% HR
Rest 3 minutes
2 × 60 yards shuttle at 70–80% HR
Use recovery heart rate of approximately 130 bpm

Cooldown

2 × walk 50 yards, jog 50 yards, RPE 4
Stretch as needed

Week 4, Day 6

Optional cardio day; same routine as Day 3

Week 5, Day 1

General Warm-Up	Jog 440 yards or spend 5 minutes on a stationary device, RPE 4
	Stretch lower body
Specific Warm-Up	Skip, hip, carioca, butt kicks, backward run
SIDs, RPE 5	1 set each, 20 yards; walk back after each
	Quick feet, 10 yards, 2 sets; walk back after each
	Skip, hip, strides, 1 power transition, 30 yards
Buildups, RPE 6	2 sets, 120 yards (40-40-40)
Energy System	2 × 100 yards at 7 RPE; walk back after each
Management (Sprints)	4 × 60 yards at 8 RPE; walk back after each
	4 × 40 yards at 8 RPE; walk back after each
	2 × 20 yards at near max; walk back after each
	Use recovery heart rate of approximately 120 bpm
Cooldown	2 × walk 50 yards, jog 50 yards, RPE 4
	Stretch upper body
Chest and Back	
Barbell chest press	4 sets, 6–8 reps, wt. _____
One arm bent-over row	4 sets, 6–8 reps, wt. _____
Shoulders	
Front shoulder flexion	3 sets, 8–10 reps, wt. _____
Side deltoid raise	3 sets, 8–10 reps, wt. _____
Rear deltoid row	3 sets, 10–12 reps, wt. _____
Rotator Cuff	
Internal rotation	2 sets, 25 reps, wt. _____
External rotation	2 sets, 25 reps, wt. _____

Arms

Biceps curl	3 sets, 6–8 reps, wt. _____
Triceps pressdown	3 sets, 6–8 reps, wt. _____

Pelvic Stabilizers

Upper trunk flexion	2 sets, 25 reps
Seated rotation	2 sets, 20 reps
Back raise	2 sets, 20 reps

Week 5, Day 2

General Warm-Up   Jog 440 yards or spend 5 minutes on a stationary device, RPE 4
Stretch lower body

Pelvic Stabilizers

Lower trunk flexion	2 sets, 20–25 reps
Seated rotation	2 sets, 20 reps
Aquaman	2 sets, 20–25 reps

Hips

Hip adduction	2 sets, 8–10 reps, wt. _____
Hip abduction	2 sets, 8–10 reps, wt. _____

Legs

Leg press	3 sets, 6–8 reps, wt. _____
Hamstring curl	3 sets, 6–8 reps, wt. _____
Walking lunge	2 sets, 15–20 reps, wt. _____
Bridge, double leg	2 sets, 15–20 reps, wt. _____
Calf raise	1 set to fatigue; 1 set for each of 3 positions

General Warm-Up   Jog 440 yards or spend 5 minutes on a stationary device, RPE 4
Stretch lower body

Specific Warm-Up   Skip, hip, carioca, butt kicks, backward run

SIDs, RPE 5   1 set each, 20 yards; walk back after each

Quick feet, 10 yards, 2 sets; walk back after each

Skip, hip, strides, 1 power transition, 30 yards

Energy System Management (Sprints)	2 × 220 yards at 70–80% HR; walk back after each Rest at least 2 minutes 2 × 150 yards at 70–80% HR; walk back after each Rest at least 2 minutes 2 × 100 yards at 70–80% HR; walk back after each Use recovery heart rate of approximately 130 bpm
Cooldown	2 × walk 50 yards, jog 50 yards, RPE 4 Stretch as needed

Week 5, Day 3

Optional Cardio Day

General Warm-Up	Jog 440 yards or spend 5 minutes on a stationary device, RPE 4 Stretch lower body
Specific Warm-Up	Stretch upper body
Pelvic Stabilizers	
Upper trunk flexion	2 sets, 25 reps
Seated rotation	2 sets, 20 reps
Back raise	2 sets, 20 reps
Cardiovascular Stationary Device	22 minutes on bike, stepper, or other device Stretch hip flexors
Cooldown	2 × walk 50 yards, jog 50 yards, RPE 4 Stretch lower body
Pelvic Stabilizers	
Lower trunk flexion	2 sets, 20–25 reps
Seated rotation	2 sets, 20 reps
Aquaman	2 sets, 20–25 reps

Week 5, Day 4

General Warm-Up	Jog 440 yards or spend 5 minutes on a stationary device, RPE 4
	Stretch lower body
Specific Warm-Up	Skip, hip, carioca, butt kicks, backward run
SIDs, RPE 5	1 set each, 20 yards; walk back after each
	Quick feet, 10 yards, 2 sets; walk back after each
	Skip, hip, strides, 1 power transition, 30 yards
Buildups, RPE 6	2 sets, 120 yards (40-40-40)
Energy System	2 × 60 yards at 7 RPE; walk back after each
Management (Sprints)	4 × 40 yards at 8 RPE; walk back after each
	4 × 20 yards at near max; walk back after each
	2 × 10 yards at near max; walk back after each
	Use recovery heart rate of approximately 120 bpm
Cooldown	2 × walk 50 yards, jog 50 yards, RPE 4
	Stretch upper body

Chest and Back

Incline chest press	4 sets, 6–8 reps, wt. _____
Lat pulldown	4 sets, 6–8 reps, wt. _____

Shoulders

Front shoulder flexion	3 sets, 8–10 reps, wt. _____
Side deltoid raise	3 sets, 8–10 reps, wt. _____
Rear deltoid row	3 sets, 10–12 reps, wt. _____

Rotator Cuff

Internal rotation	2 sets, 25 to fatigue, wt. _____
External rotation	2 sets, 25 to fatigue, wt. _____

Arms

Alternating biceps curl	3 sets, 6–8 reps, wt. _____
Dumbbell triceps extension	3 sets, 6–8 reps, wt. _____

Pelvic Stabilizers

Upper trunk flexion	2 sets, 25 reps
Seated rotation	2 sets, 20 reps
Back raise	2 sets, 20 reps

Week 5, Day 5

General Warm-Up
Jog 440 yards or spend 5 minutes on a stationary device, RPE 4
Stretch lower body

Pelvic Stabilizers

Lower trunk flexion	2 sets, 20–25 reps
Seated rotation	2 sets, 20 reps
Aquaman	2 sets, 20–25 reps

Hips

Hip adduction	2 sets, 8–10 reps, wt. _____
Hip abduction	2 sets, 8–10 reps, wt. _____

Legs

Leg press	3 sets, 6–8 reps, wt. _____
Hamstring curl	3 sets, 6–8 reps, wt. _____
Walking lunge	2 sets, 15–20 reps, wt. _____
Bridge, double leg	2 sets, 15–20 reps, wt. _____
Calf raise	1 set to fatigue; 1 set for each of 3 positions

General Warm-Up
Jog 440 yards or spend 5 minutes on a stationary device, RPE 4
Stretch lower body

Specific Warm-Up
Jump rope at major league level

**Energy System Management
(Shuttles and Half-Gasser)**
2×60 yard shuttle at 70–80% HR
$2 \times$ half-gasser at 70–80% HR
Rest 2 minutes between each
Use recovery heart rate of approximately 130 bpm

Cooldown	2 × walk 50 yards, jog 50 yards, RPE 4
	Stretch as needed

Week 5, Day 6

Optional cardio day; same routine as Day 3

Week 6, Day 1

General Warm-Up	Jog 440 yards or spend 5 minutes on a stationary device, RPE 4
	Stretch lower body
Specific Warm-Up	Skip, hip, carioca, butt kicks, backward run
SIDs, RPE 5	1 set each, 20 yards; walk back after each
	Quick feet, 10 yards, 2 sets; walk back after each
	Skip, hip, strides, 1 power transition, 30 yards
Buildups, RPE 6	2 sets, 120 yards (40-40-40)
Energy System Management (Sprints)	2 × 100 yards at 7 RPE; walk back after each
	4 × 60 yards at 8 RPE; walk back after each
	4 × 40 yards at 8 RPE; walk back after each
	2 × 20 yards at near max; walk back after each
	Use recovery heart rate of approximately 120 bpm
Cooldown	2 × walk 50 yards, jog 50 yards, RPE 4
	Stretch upper body
Chest and Back	
Barbell chest press	4 sets, 6–8 reps, wt. _____
One arm bent-over row	4 sets, 6–8 reps, wt. _____
Shoulders	
Front shoulder flexion	3 sets, 8–10 reps, wt. _____
Side deltoid raise	3 sets, 8–10 reps, wt. _____
Rear deltoid row	3 sets, 10–12 reps, wt. _____

Rotator Cuff

Internal rotation	2 sets, 25 reps, wt. _____
External rotation	2 sets, 25 reps, wt. _____

Arms

Biceps curl	3 sets, 6–8 reps, wt. _____
Triceps pressdown	3 sets, 6–8 reps, wt. _____

Pelvic Stabilizers

Upper trunk flexion	2 sets, 25 reps
Seated rotation	2 sets, 20 reps
Back raise	2 sets, 20 reps

Week 6, Day 2

General Warm-Up

Jog 440 yards or spend 5 minutes on a stationary device, RPE 4
Stretch lower body

Pelvic Stabilizers

Lower trunk flexion	2 sets, 20–25 reps
Seated rotation	2 sets, 20 reps
Aquaman	2 sets, 20–25 reps

Hips

Hip adduction	2 sets, 8–10 reps, wt. _____
Hip abduction	2 sets, 8–10 reps, wt. _____

Legs

Leg press	3 sets, 6–8 reps, wt. _____
Hamstring curl	3 sets, 6–8 reps, wt. _____
Walking lunge	2 sets, 15–20 reps, wt. _____
Bridge, double leg	2 sets, 15–20 reps, wt. _____
Calf raise	1 set to fatigue; 1 set for each of 3 positions

General Warm-Up

Jog 440 yards or spend 5 minutes on a stationary device, RPE 4
Stretch lower body

Specific Warm-Up	Skip, hip, carioca, butt kicks, backward run
SIDs, RPE 5	1 set each, 20 yards; walk back after each
	Quick feet, 10 yards, 2 sets; walk back after each
	Skip, hip, strides, 1 power transition, 30 yards
Energy System	2 × 220 yards at 70–80% HR; walk back after each
Management (Sprints)	Rest at least 2 minutes
	3 × 150 yards at 70–80% HR; walk back after each
	Rest at least 2 minutes
	3 × 100 yards at 70–80% HR; walk back after each
	Use recovery heart rate of approximately 130 bpm
Cooldown	2 × walk 50 yards, jog 50 yards, RPE 4
	Stretch as needed

Week 6, Day 3

Optional Cardio Day

General Warm-Up	Jog 440 yards or spend 5 minutes on a stationary device, RPE 4
	Stretch lower body
Specific Warm-Up	Stretch upper body
Pelvic Stabilizers	
Upper trunk flexion	2 sets, 25 reps
Seated rotation	2 sets, 20 reps
Back raise	2 sets, 20 reps
Cardiovascular	24 minutes on bike, stepper, or other device
Stationary Device	Stretch hip flexors
Cooldown	2 × walk 50 yards, jog 50 yards, RPE 4
	Stretch lower body
Pelvic Stabilizers	
Lower trunk flexion	2 sets, 20–25 reps
Seated rotation	2 sets, 20 reps
Aquaman	2 sets, 20–25 reps

Week 6, Day 4

General Warm-Up	Jog 440 yards or spend 5 minutes on a stationary device, RPE 4
	Stretch lower body

Specific Warm-Up	Skip, hip, carioca, butt kicks, backward run
SIDs, RPE 5	1 set each, 20 yards; walk back after each
	Quick feet, 10 yards, 2 sets; walk back after each
	Skip, hip, strides, 1 power transition, 30 yards
Buildups, RPE 6	2 sets, 120 yards (40-40-40)

Energy System	2×60 yards at 7 RPE; walk back after each
Management (Sprints)	4×40 yards at 8 RPE; walk back after each
	4×20 yards at near max; walk back after each
	4×10 yards at near max; walk back after each
	Use recovery heart rate of approximately 120 bpm

Cooldown	$2 \times$ walk 50 yards, jog 50 yards, RPE 4
	Stretch upper body

Chest and Back

Incline chest press	4 sets, 6–8 reps, wt. _____
Lat pulldown	4 sets, 6–8 reps, wt. _____

Shoulders

Front shoulder flexion	3 sets, 8–10 reps, wt. _____
Side deltoid raise	3 sets, 8–10 reps, wt. _____
Rear deltoid row	3 sets, 10–12 reps, wt. _____

Rotator Cuff

Internal rotation	2 sets, 25 to fatigue, wt. _____
External rotation	2 sets, 25 to fatigue, wt. _____

Arms

Alternating biceps curl	3 sets, 6–8 reps, wt. _____
Dumbbell triceps extension	3 sets, 6–8 reps, wt. _____

Pelvic Stabilizers

Upper trunk flexion	2 sets, 25 reps
Seated rotation	2 sets, 20 reps
Back raise	2 sets, 20 reps

Week 6, Day 5

General Warm-Up

Jog 440 yards or spend 5 minutes on a stationary device, RPE 4
Stretch lower body

Pelvic Stabilizers

Lower trunk flexion	2 sets, 20–25 reps
Seated rotation	2 sets, 20 reps
Aquaman	2 sets, 20–25 reps

Hips

Hip adduction	2 sets, 8–10 reps, wt. _____
Hip abduction	2 sets, 8–10 reps, wt. _____

Legs

Leg press	3 sets, 6–8 reps, wt. _____
Hamstring curl	3 sets, 6–8 reps, wt. _____
Walking lunge	2 sets, 15–20 reps, wt. _____
Bridge, double leg	2 sets, 15–20 reps, wt. _____
Calf raise	1 set to fatigue; 1 set for each of 3 positions

General Warm-Up

Jog 440 yards or spend 5 minutes on a stationary device, RPE 4
Stretch lower body

Specific Warm-Up

Jump rope at major league level

Energy System Management (Shuttles and Half-Gasser)

1×100 yard shuttle at 70–80% HR
1×60 yard shuttle at 70–80% HR
$1 \times$ half-gasser at 70–80% HR
Rest $1\frac{1}{2}$ minutes between each
Use recovery heart rate of approximately 130 bpm

Cooldown	2 × walk 50 yards, jog 50 yards, RPE 4
	Stretch as needed

Week 6, Day 6

Optional cardio day; same routine as Day 3

The Maintenance Program

This program is designed to help you to maintain your muscle gains. If you get bored, you may wish to work with a trainer from time to time to develop different exercises to work the same muscle groups.

Maintenance Program, Day 1

General Warm-Up	Jog 440 yards or spend 5 minutes on a stationary device, RPE 4
	Stretch lower body
Specific Warm-Up	Skip, hip, carioca, butt kicks, backward run
SIDs, RPE 5	1 set each, 20 yards; walk back after each
	Quick feet, 10 yards, 2 sets; walk back after each
	Skip, hip, strides, 1 power transition, 30 yards
Buildups, RPE 6	2 sets, 120 yards (40-40-40)
Energy System	2 × 100 yards at 7 RPE; walk back after each
Management (Sprints)	4 × 60 yards at 8 RPE; walk back after each
	4 × 40 yards at 8 RPE; walk back after each
	2 × 20 yards at near max; walk back after each
	Use recovery heart rate of approximately 120 bpm
Cooldown	2 × walk 50 yards, jog 50 yards, RPE 4
	Stretch upper body
Chest and Back	
Barbell chest press	4 sets, 6–8 reps, wt. _____
One arm bent-over row	4 sets, 6–8 reps, wt. _____

Shoulders

Front shoulder flexion	3 sets, 8–10 reps, wt. _____
Side deltoid raise	3 sets, 8–10 reps, wt. _____
Rear deltoid row	3 sets, 10–12 reps, wt. _____

Rotator Cuff

Internal rotation	2 sets, 25 reps, wt. _____
External rotation	2 sets, 25 reps, wt. _____

Arms

Biceps curl	3 sets, 6–8 reps, wt. _____
Triceps pressdown	3 sets, 6–8 reps, wt. _____

Pelvic Stabilizers

Upper trunk flexion	2 sets, 25 reps
Seated rotation	2 sets, 20 reps
Back raise	2 sets, 20 reps

Maintenance Program, Day 2

General Warm-Up   Jog 440 yards or spend 5 minutes on a stationary device, RPE 4
Stretch lower body

Pelvic Stabilizers

Lower trunk flexion	2 sets, 20–25 reps
Seated rotation	2 sets, 20 reps
Aquaman	2 sets, 20–25 reps

Hips

Hip adduction	2 sets, 8–10 reps, wt. _____
Hip abduction	2 sets, 8–10 reps, wt. _____

Legs

Leg press	3 sets, 6–8 reps, wt. _____
Hamstring curl	3 sets, 6–8 reps, wt. _____

Walking lunge	2 sets, 15–20 reps, wt. _____
Bridge, double leg	2 sets, 15–20 reps, wt. _____
Calf raise	1 set to fatigue; 1 set for each of 3 positions

General Warm-Up

Jog 440 yards or spend 5 minutes on a stationary device, RPE 4

Stretch lower body

Specific Warm-Up

SIDs, RPE 5

Skip, hip, carioca, butt kicks, backward run

1 set each, 20 yards; walk back after each

Quick feet, 10 yards, 2 sets; walk back after each

Skip, hip, strides, 1 power transition, 30 yards

Energy System Management (Sprints)

2 × 220 yards at 70–80% HR; walk back after each

Rest at least 2 minutes

3 × 150 yards at 70–80% HR; walk back after each

Rest at least 2 minutes

3 × 100 yards at 70–80% HR; walk back after each

Use recovery heart rate of approximately 130 bpm

Cooldown

2 × walk 50 yards, jog 50 yards, RPE 4

Stretch as needed

Maintenance Program, Day 3

Optional Cardio Day

General Warm-Up

Jog 440 yards or spend 5 minutes on a stationary device, RPE 4

Stretch lower body

Specific Warm-Up

Stretch upper body

Pelvic Stabilizers

Upper trunk flexion	2 sets, 25 reps
Seated rotation	2 sets, 20 reps
Back raise	2 sets, 20 reps

Cardiovascular Stationary Device

24 minutes on bike, stepper, or other device

Stretch hip flexors

| **Cooldown** | 2 × walk 50 yards, jog 50 yards, RPE 4 |
| | Stretch lower body |

Pelvic Stabilizers

Lower trunk flexion	2 sets, 20–25 reps
Seated rotation	2 sets, 20 reps
Aquaman	2 sets, 20–25 reps

Maintenance Program, Day 4

| **General Warm-Up** | Jog 440 yards or spend 5 minutes on a stationary device, RPE 4 |
| | Stretch lower body |

Chest and Back

| Incline chest press | 4 sets, 6–8 reps, wt. _____ |
| Lat pulldown | 4 sets, 6–8 reps, wt. _____ |

Shoulders

Front shoulder flexion	3 sets, 8–10 reps, wt. _____
Side deltoid raise	3 sets, 8–10 reps, wt. _____
Rear deltoid row	3 sets, 10–12 reps, wt. _____

Rotator Cuff

| Internal rotation | 2 sets, 25 reps to fatigue, wt. _____ |
| External rotation | 2 sets, 25 reps to fatigue, wt. _____ |

Arms

| Alternating biceps curl | 3 sets, 6–8 reps, wt. _____ |
| Dumbbell triceps extension | 3 sets, 6–8 reps, wt. _____ |

Pelvic Stabilizers

Upper trunk flexion	2 sets, 25 reps
Lower trunk flexion	2 sets, 20–25 reps
Seated rotation	2 sets, 20 reps
Back raise	2 sets, 20 reps
Aquaman	2 sets, 20 reps

Hips

Hip adduction	2 sets, 8–10 reps, wt. _____
Hip abduction	2 sets, 8–10 reps, wt. _____

Legs

Leg press	3 sets, 6–8 reps, wt. _____
Hamstring curl	3 sets, 6–8 reps, wt. _____
Walking lunge	2 sets, 15–20 reps, wt. _____
Bridge, double leg	2 sets, 15–20 reps, wt. _____
Calf raise	1 set to fatigue; 1 set for each of 3 positions

Cooldown 2 × walk 50 yards, jog 50 yards, RPE 4
Stretch as needed

Maintenance Program, Day 5

General Warm-Up Jog 440 yards or spend 5 minutes on a stationary device, RPE 4
Stretch lower body

Specific Warm-Up Jump rope at major league level

Energy System Management (Shuttles and Half-Gasser)
1 × 100 yards shuttle at 70%–80% HR
1 × 60 yards shuttle at 70–80% HR
1 × half-gasser at 70–80% HR
Rest 1½ minutes between each
Use recovery heart rate of approximately 130 bpm

Cooldown 2 × walk 50 yards, jog 50 yards, RPE 4
Stretch as needed

Maintenance Program, Day 6

Optional cardio day; same routine as Day 3

PART FOUR

Your Daily Muscle-Building Guide

12

The Lean and Hard
Workout Program Guide

This chapter serves as a guide to help you successfully accomplish your twenty-four muscle-building workouts and to keep track of your high-performance nutrition and supplementation. You should begin to notice significant changes in your energy levels, strength, and appearance after only two weeks.

While no one ever follows a program perfectly, remember that the greater your compliance with the Lean and Hard Program, the greater your gains in muscle and the lower your body fat will become. Strive to improve your faithfulness to the program every workout day. Remember, twenty-four high-intensity workouts over six weeks is a small price to pay for an average gain of 10 pounds of lean muscle and an average loss of 6 pounds of body fat.

Here are a few things to remember:

- Never take your physician out of the loop. He or she must be consulted before, during, and after your program, just as we do in my sports program. This is a team effort.
- It takes nutritional support to build lean muscle. Eating your three main meals and three snacks daily will give your body the nutrients and energy it needs to support your high-intensity workout and repair and build muscle between workouts.
- The timing of taking your supplements is vitally important. Try to always take your high-performance supplementation—whey protein, L-glutamine, creatine monohydrate, and maltodextrin—on schedule. The supplementation guidelines I have set up in this book are designed to minimize muscle

breakdown and maximize muscle building, plus give you the energy you need for high performance.

- Don't skip warm-ups and cooldowns. The stretching routines, walks, and drills I give you are specifically designed to prepare your body for your HIT workout and to help you recover between each segment of your workout.

- Perform your high-intensity workout warm-ups, drills, and exercises in the order in which they are given. Follow your workout guide *exactly* if you wish to get maximum results. Strive to do all of the repetitions and sets indicated for each exercise. If you find you cannot finish the specified reps, decrease the weight you are using slightly, by 5 pounds or so, until you can.

- Try to increase your weights by 5 pounds or so each week. Keep challenging your body so that your muscle gain continues to increase rapidly.

- Always work out smart. Remember what I taught you in chapter 1: don't think that you will get greater results by performing high-intensity training six or seven days a week. Your recovery days play a *vitally important* role in your body's ability to build lean muscle.

Calculating Your Body's Muscle-to-Fat Percentage

Before you begin the Lean and Hard HIT Program, you may wish to evaluate your percentage of lean tissue to body fat so that you can measure how much muscle you have gained by the end of your twenty-four workouts. You may choose to have your body composition measured by a professional at your local gym or YMCA, but here is a simple at-home test to give you a fairly accurate idea of where you stand. This test is slightly different for males and females, and I have included both versions below.

You do not necessarily have to get your body fat tested to know that your body composition is improving. If you have been performing your exercises properly and staying faithful to your high-performance nutrition and supplementation schedules, your clothes should begin to feel looser. If you find yourself taking in your belt a notch or two or if you observe increased strength, you will know that you are losing fat and gaining lean muscle.

At-Home Body-Fat Test for Males

Step 1: Take Your Measurements

1. Height in inches _____
2. Hips in inches _____
3. Waist in inches _____
4. Weight in pounds _____

Step 2: Determine Your Percentage of Body Fat

1. Multiply your hips (inches) ___ × 1.4 = ___ – 2 = ___ (A)
2. Multiply your waist (inches) ___ × 0.72 = ___ – 4 = ___ (B)
3. Add A + B = ___ (C)
4. Multiply your height (inches) ___ × 0.61 = ___ (D)
5. Subtract D from C, then subtract 10 more: C – D – 10 = _____ % fat

Your answer will be your approximate body fat percentage.

At-Home Body-Fat Test for Females

Step 1: Take Your Measurements

1. Height in inches _____
2. Hips in inches _____
3. Waist in inches _____
4. Weight in pounds _____

Step 2: Determine Your Percentage of Body Fat

1. Multiply your hips (inches) ___ × 1.4 = ___ – 1 = ___ (A)
2. Multiply your waist (inches) ___ × 0.72 = ___ – 2 = ___ (B)
3. Add A + B = ___ (C)
4. Multiply your height (inches) ___ × 0.61 = ___ (D)
5. Subtract D from C, then subtract 10 more: C – D – 10 = _____ % fat

Your answer will be your approximate body fat percentage.

Calculating Your Pounds of Lean Muscle vs. Body Fat

The final step is to take your total weight and calculate how many pounds of fat and how many pounds of lean muscle you carry. To do so, use the following two formulas:

Total weight (pounds) × percent body fat = total pounds of fat

Total weight – total pounds of fat = total pounds of lean muscle

For example, if you are a woman weighing 150 pounds and you find that you have 30 percent body fat, you would calculate the number of pounds of fat you carry using the following formula:

$$150 \text{ lb.} \times .30 \text{ (percent body fat)} = 45 \text{ lb. of fat}$$

To calculate your pounds of lean muscle, you would use the following formula:

$$150 \text{ lb.} - 45 \text{ lb. of fat} = 105 \text{ lb. of lean muscle}$$

I suggest reevaluating your lean tissue to fat percentage every three weeks. To help you understand the meaning of your body composition, here is a chart that defines healthy and unhealthy body fat percentages for men and women.

BODY FAT PERCENTAGE

Level	Men	Women
Excellent, very lean	<11	<14
Good/lean	11–14	14–17
Average	15–17	18–22
Fair/fat	18–22	23–27
Obese	22+	27+

Lean and Hard Training Program Logs

I'd like you to photocopy the following checklist. Take a moment at the end of each workout day to check off each statement with a plus (+) or a minus (−). Your ultimate goal is perfect compliance.

High-Intensity Training Checklist

I ate three nutritious meals and two or three snacks _____

I chose only lean protein sources _____

I chose complex carbohydrates over simple sugars _____

I had at least five servings of vegetables _____

I had at least two servings of fruit _____

I limited saturated fats and ate healthy unsaturated fats _____

I drank between ½ and 1 ounce of water per pound of body weight _____

I did not have more than two cups of coffee or tea _____

I avoided soft drinks containing sugar and caffeine _____

I did not allow more than three or four hours between meals and snacks _____

I understand that desserts are a special treat, so I skipped mine _____

I did not eat after eight at night _____

I took my performance nutritional supplements on schedule _____

I warmed up before exercising _____

I did all of my stretching routines, drills, and exercises in the order indicated _____

I used the proper rate of perceive exertion (RPE) _____

I allowed my heart rate (HR) to return to the prescribed beats per minute (bpm) _____

I performed my designated cooldown routine _____

I increased my weights every week _____

Daily Program

Week 1, Day 1

High-Performance Nutrition

Use the guidelines for high-performance nutrition in chapters 3 through 5. Also include what *time* you eat each meal.

Breakfast _____

Snack _____

Lunch _____

Snack _____

Dinner _____

Snack _____

Daily fluid intake _____
(Aim for ½ to 1 ounce per pound of body weight. Example: if you weigh 160 pounds, you should drink between one and a half and three 1.5 liter bottles of water.)

Coffee, tea, sodas _____
(Always drink these in moderation since they contain caffeine and sugar. Most of your daily fluid intake should be water.)

High-performance Nutrition Supplementation

Following the guidelines in chapters 6 and 7, check off the items that apply.

I took my prebreakfast loading dose of creatine monohydrate _____

I took my preworkout supplements _____

I stayed hydrated during my workout _____

I took my postworkout supplements _____

I took my loading doses of creatine monohydrate pre- and postworkout and before two meals _____

I took my multivitamins/minerals and antioxidants on schedule _____

Daily Exercise

Following the guidelines in chapters 8 through 11, check off the items that apply.

I performed my general warm-up and stretching routine at the proper rate of perceived exertion (RPE) _____

I performed my specific warm-up at the proper RPE _____

I performed my energy system management exercises at the proper RPE _____

I allowed my heart rate (HR) to recover to 120 beats per minute (bpm) _____

I performed my cooldown at the proper RPE _____

I performed my upper-body exercises in the order indicated _____

I completed all my sets and reps _____ Amount of weight used _____

How I felt at the end of my workout _____

Week 1, Day 2

High-Performance Nutrition

Use the guidelines for high-performance nutrition in chapters 3 through 5. Also include what *time* you eat each meal.

Breakfast _____

Snack _____

Lunch _____

Snack _____

Dinner _____

Snack _____

Daily fluid intake _____
(Aim for ½ to 1 ounce per pound of body weight. Example: if you weigh 160 pounds, you should drink between one and a half and three 1.5 liter bottles of water.)

Coffee, tea, sodas _____
(Always drink these in moderation since they contain caffeine and sugar. Most of your daily fluid intake should be water.)

High-performance Nutrition Supplementation

Following the guidelines in chapters 6 and 7, check off the items that apply.

I took my prebreakfast loading dose of creatine monohydrate _____

I took my preworkout supplements _____

I stayed hydrated during my workout _____

I took my postworkout supplements _____

I took my loading doses of creatine monohydrate pre- and postworkout and before two meals _____

I took my multivitamins/minerals and antioxidants on schedule _____

Daily Exercise

Following the guidelines in chapters 8 through 11, check off the items that apply.

I performed my general warm-up and stretching routine at the proper RPE

_____

I performed my pelvic stabilizer exercises in the order indicated _____

I performed my lower body exercises in the order indicated _____

I completed all my sets and reps _____ Amount of weight used _____

I performed my general warm-up at the proper RPE _____

I performed my specific warm-up at the proper RPE _____

I performed my energy system management exercises at the proper RPE _____

I allowed my HR to recover to 120 bpm _____

I performed my cooldown at the proper RPE _____

How I felt at the end of my workout _____

Week 1, Day 3

Optional Cardio Day

Since this is the week when you are taking your loading doses of creatine monohydrate, if you do not do a cardio workout on this day, still take 20 g of creatine monohydrate, divided into four doses, throughout the day.

High-Performance Nutrition

Use the guidelines for high-performance nutrition in chapters 3 through 5. Also include what *time* you eat each meal.

Breakfast _____

Snack _____

Lunch _____

Snack _____

Dinner _____

Snack _____

Daily fluid intake _____
(Aim for $\frac{1}{2}$ to 1 ounce per pound of body weight. Example: if you weigh 160 pounds, you should drink between one and a half and three 1.5 liter bottles of water.)

Coffee, tea, sodas _____
(Always drink these in moderation since they contain caffeine and sugar. Most of your daily fluid intake should be water.)

High-performance Nutrition Supplementation

Following the guidelines in chapters 6 and 7, check off the items that apply.

I took my prebreakfast loading dose of creatine monohydrate _____

I took my preworkout supplements _____

I stayed hydrated during my workout _____

I took my postworkout supplements _____

I took my loading doses of creatine monohydrate pre- and postworkout and before two meals _____

I took my multivitamins/minerals and antioxidants on schedule _____

If this is a nonworkout day, take only the creatine monohydrate as:

   1 serving prebreakfast _____

   1 serving prelunch _____

   1 serving predinner _____

   1 serving presleep (only on Day 3, which is a creatine-loading day) _____

Daily Exercise

Remember, this routine is optional. Following the guidelines in chapters 8 through 11, check off the items that apply.

I performed my general warm-up and stretching routine at the proper RPE _____

I performed my specific warm-up (stretches) at the proper RPE _____

I performed my pelvic stabilizer exercises in the order indicated _____

I completed all my sets and reps _____ Amount of weight used _____

I performed my cardiovascular exercise _____

I performed my cooldown routine at the proper RPE _____

I performed my second set of pelvic stabilizers in the order indicated _____

I performed all my sets and reps _____ (no weights required)

How I felt at the end of my workout _____

_____ Week 1, Day 4 _____

High-Performance Nutrition

Use the guidelines for high-performance nutrition in chapters 3 through 5. Also include what *time* you eat each meal.

Breakfast _____

Snack _____

Lunch _____

Snack _____

Dinner _____

Snack _____

Daily fluid intake _____
(Aim for ½ to 1 ounce per pound of body weight. Example: if you weigh 160 pounds, you should drink between one and a half and three 1.5 liter bottles of water.)

Coffee, tea, sodas _____
(Always drink these in moderation since they contain caffeine and sugar. Most of your daily fluid intake should be water.)

High-Performance Nutrition Supplementation

Following the guidelines in chapters 6 and 7, check off the items that apply.

I took my preworkout supplements _____

I stayed hydrated during my workout _____

I took my postworkout supplements _____

I took my presleep supplements _____

I took my multivitamins/minerals and antioxidants on schedule _____

Daily Exercise

Following the guidelines in chapters 8 through 11, check off the items that apply.

I performed my general warm-up and stretching routine at the proper RPE
_____

I performed my specific warm-up routine at the proper RPE _____

I performed my energy system management exercises at the proper RPE ____

I allowed my HR to recover to 120 bpm ____

I performed my cooldown at the proper RPE ____

I performed my upper body exercises in the order indicated ____

I completed all my sets and reps ____ Amount of weight used ____

I performed my pelvic stabilizers in the order indicated ____

I performed the required sets and repetitions (weights not used) ____

How I felt at the end of my workout _____

Week 1, Day 5

High-Performance Nutrition

Use the guidelines for high-performance nutrition in chapters 3 through 5. Also include what *time* you eat each meal.

Breakfast _____

Snack _____

Lunch _____

Snack _____

Dinner _____

Snack _____

Daily fluid intake _____
(Aim for ½ to 1 ounce per pound of body weight. Example: if you weigh 160 pounds, you should drink between one and a half and three 1.5 liter bottles of water.)

Coffee, tea, sodas _____
(Always drink these in moderation since they contain caffeine and sugar. Most of your daily fluid intake should be water.)

High-Performance Nutrition Supplementation

Following the guidelines in chapters 6 and 7, check off the items that apply.

I took my preworkout supplements ____

I stayed hydrated during my workout ____

I took my postworkout supplements ____

I took my multivitamins/minerals and antioxidants on schedule ____

Daily Exercise

Following the guidelines in chapters 8 through 11, check off the items that apply.

I performed my general warm-up and stretching routine at the proper RPE
____

I performed my pelvic stabilizer exercises in the order indicated ____

I performed my lower body exercises in the order indicated ____

I completed all my sets and reps ____ Amount of weight used ____

I performed my general warm-up at the proper RPE ____

I performed my specific warm-up at the proper RPE ____

I performed my energy system management exercises at the proper RPE ____

I allowed my HR to recover to 130 bpm ____

I performed my cooldown at the proper RPE ____

I stretched as needed ____

How I felt at the end of my workout _____

Week 1, Day 6

Optional Cardio Day

High-Performance Nutrition

Use the guidelines for high-performance nutrition in chapters 3 through 5. Also include what *time* you eat each meal.

Breakfast _____

Snack _____

Lunch _____

Snack _____

Dinner _____

Snack _____

Daily fluid intake _____
(Aim for ½ to 1 ounce per pound of body weight. Example: if you weigh 160 pounds, you should drink between one and a half and three 1.5 liter bottles of water.)

Coffee, tea, sodas _____
(Always drink these in moderation since they contain caffeine and sugar. Most of your daily fluid intake should be water.)

High-Performance Nutrition Supplementation

No supplementation unless you make this your optional cardio day. In that case, follow the Wednesday supplementation schedule on page 106.

Daily Exercise

Remember, this routine is optional. Following the guidelines in chapters 8 through 11, check off the items that apply.

I performed my general warm-up and stretching routine at the proper RPE

_____

I performed my specific warm-up (stretches) at the proper RPE _____

I performed my pelvic stabilizer exercises in the order indicated _____

I completed all my sets and reps _____ Amount of weight used _____

I performed my cardiovascular exercise _____

I performed my cooldown routine at the proper RPE _____

I performed my second set of pelvic stabilizers in the order indicated _____

I performed all my sets and reps _____ (no weights required)

How I felt at the end of my workout _____

Week 1, Day 7

Rest and Recovery Day

High-Performance Nutrition

Use the guidelines for high-performance nutrition in chapters 3 through 5. Also include what *time* you eat each meal.

Breakfast _____

Snack _____

Lunch _____

Snack _____

Dinner _____

Snack _____

Daily fluid intake _____
(Aim for ½ to 1 ounce per pound of body weight. Example: if you weigh 160 pounds, you should drink between one and a half and three 1.5 liter bottles of water.)

Coffee, tea, sodas _____

(Always drink these in moderation since they contain caffeine and sugar. Most of your daily fluid intake should be water.)

High-Performance Nutrition Supplementation

No supplementation.

No Exercise

Make this a true rest-and-recovery day. This practice will greatly enhance your body's energy and muscle-building capacity. See chapter 1 for the reasons behind taking rest-and-recovery days.

Week 2, Day 1

High-Performance Nutrition

Use the guidelines for high-performance nutrition in chapters 3 through 5. Also include what *time* you eat each meal.

Breakfast _____

Snack _____

Lunch _____

Snack _____

Dinner _____

Snack _____

Daily fluid intake _____
(Aim for ½ to 1 ounce per pound of body weight. Example: if you weigh 160 pounds, you should drink between one and a half and three 1.5 liter bottles of water.)

Coffee, tea, sodas _____
(Always drink these in moderation since they contain caffeine and sugar. Most of your daily fluid intake should be water.)

High-Performance Nutrition Supplementation

Following the guidelines in chapters 6 and 7, check off the items that apply.

I took my preworkout supplements _____

I stayed hydrated during my workout _____

I took my postworkout supplements _____

I took my presleep supplements _____

I took my multivitamins/minerals and antioxidants on schedule _____

Daily Exercise

Following the guidelines in chapters 8 through 11, check off the items that apply.

I performed my general warm-up and stretching routine at the proper rate of
perceived exertion (RPE) _____

I performed my specific warm-up at the proper RPE _____

I performed my energy system management exercises at the proper RPE _____

I allowed my heart rate (HR) to recover to 120 beats per minute (bpm) _____

I performed my cooldown at the proper RPE _____

I performed my upper-body exercises in the order indicated _____

I completed all my sets and reps _____ Amount of weight used _____

How I felt at the end of my workout _____

Week 2, Day 2

High-Performance Nutrition

Use the guidelines for high-performance nutrition in chapters 3 through 5.
Also include what *time* you eat each meal.

Breakfast _____

Snack _____

Lunch _____

Snack _____

Dinner _____

Snack _____

Daily fluid intake _____
(Aim for ½ to 1 ounce per pound of body weight. Example: if you weigh 160
pounds, you should drink between one and a half and three 1.5 liter bottles
of water.)

Coffee, tea, sodas _____
(Always drink these in moderation since they contain caffeine and sugar.
Most of your daily fluid intake should be water.)

High-Performance Nutrition Supplementation

Following the guidelines in chapters 6 and 7, check off the items that apply.

I took my preworkout supplements _____

I stayed hydrated during my workout _____

I took my postworkout supplements ____

I took my presleep supplements ____

I took my multivitamins/minerals and antioxidants on schedule ____

Daily Exercise

Following the guidelines in chapters 8 through 11, check off the items that apply.

I performed my general warm-up and stretching routine at the proper RPE

____

I performed my pelvic stabilizer exercises in the order indicated ____

I performed my lower body exercises in the order indicated ____

I completed all my sets and reps ____ Amount of weight used ____

I performed my general warm-up at the proper RPE ____

I performed my specific warm-up at the proper RPE ____

I performed my energy system management exercises at the proper RPE ____

I allowed my HR to recover to 120 bpm ____

I performed my cooldown at the proper RPE ____

How I felt at the end of my workout _____

Week 2, Day 3

Optional Cardio Day

High-Performance Nutrition

Use the guidelines for high-performance nutrition in chapters 3 through 5. Also include what *time* you eat each meal.

Breakfast _____

Snack _____

Lunch _____

Snack _____

Dinner _____

Snack _____

Daily fluid intake _____
(Aim for ½ to 1 ounce per pound of body weight. Example: if you weigh 160 pounds, you should drink between one and a half and three 1.5 liter bottles of water.)

Coffee, tea, sodas _____

(Always drink these in moderation since they contain caffeine and sugar. Most of your daily fluid intake should be water.)

High-Performance Nutrition Supplementation

Following the guidelines in chapters 6 and 7, check off the items that apply.

I took my preworkout supplements _____

I stayed hydrated during my workout _____

I took my postworkout supplements _____

I took my presleep supplements _____

I took my multivitamins/minerals and antioxidants on schedule _____

If this is a nonworkout day, take no supplementation.

Daily Exercise

Remember, this routine is optional. Following the guidelines in chapters 8 through 11, check off the items that apply.

I performed my general warm-up and stretching routine at the proper RPE _____

I performed my specific warm-up (stretches) at the proper RPE _____

I performed my pelvic stabilizer exercises in the order indicated _____

I completed all my sets and reps _____ Amount of weight used _____

I performed my cardiovascular exercise _____

I performed my cooldown routine at the proper RPE _____

I performed my second set of pelvic stabilizers in the order indicated _____

I performed all my sets and reps _____ (no weights required)

How I felt at the end of my workout _____

Week 2, Day 4

High-Performance Nutrition

Use the guidelines for high-performance nutrition in chapters 3 through 5. Also include what *time* you eat each meal.

Breakfast _____

Snack _____

Lunch _____

Snack _____

Dinner _____

Snack _____

Daily fluid intake _____
(Aim for ½ to 1 ounce per pound of body weight. Example: if you weigh 160 pounds, you should drink between one and a half and three 1.5 liter bottles of water.)

Coffee, tea, sodas _____
(Always drink these in moderation since they contain caffeine and sugar. Most of your daily fluid intake should be water.)

High-Performance Nutrition Supplementation

Following the guidelines in chapters 6 and 7, check off the items that apply.

I took my preworkout supplements ____

I stayed hydrated during my workout ____

I took my postworkout supplements ____

I took my presleep supplements ____

I took my multivitamins/minerals and antioxidants on schedule ____

Daily Exercise

Following the guidelines in chapters 8 through 11, check off the items that apply.

I performed my general warm-up and stretching routine at the proper RPE ____

I performed my specific warm-up routine at the proper RPE ____

I performed my energy system management exercises at the proper RPE ____

I allowed my HR to recover to 120 bpm ____

I performed my cooldown at the proper RPE ____

I performed my upper body exercises in the order indicated ____

I completed all my sets and reps ____ Amount of weight used ____

I performed my pelvic stabilizers in the order indicated ____

I performed the required sets and repetitions (weights not used) ____

How I felt at the end of my workout _____

Week 2, Day 5

High-Performance Nutrition

Use the guidelines for high-performance nutrition in chapters 3 through 5. Also include what *time* you eat each meal.

Breakfast _____

Snack _____

Lunch _____

Snack _____

Dinner _____

Snack _____

Daily fluid intake _____
(Aim for ½ to 1 ounce per pound of body weight. Example: if you weigh 160 pounds, you should drink between one and a half and three 1.5 liter bottles of water.)

Coffee, tea, sodas _____
(Always drink these in moderation since they contain caffeine and sugar. Most of your daily fluid intake should be water.)

High-Performance Nutrition Supplementation

Following the guidelines in chapters 6 and 7, check off the items that apply.

I took my preworkout supplements _____

I stayed hydrated during my workout _____

I took my postworkout supplements _____

I took my presleep supplements _____

I took my multivitamins/minerals and antioxidants on schedule _____

Daily Exercise

Following the guidelines in chapters 8 through 11, check off the items that apply.

I performed my general warm-up and stretching routine at the proper RPE _____

I performed my pelvic stabilizer exercises in the order indicated _____

I performed my lower body exercises in the order indicated _____

I completed all my sets and reps _____ Amount of weight used _____

I performed my general warm-up at the proper RPE _____

I performed my specific warm-up at the proper RPE _____

I performed my energy system management exercises at the proper RPE _____

I allowed my HR to recover to 130 bpm _____

I performed my cooldown at the proper RPE _____

I stretched as needed _____

How I felt at the end of my workout _____

Week 2, Day 6

Optional Cardio Day

High-Performance Nutrition

Use the guidelines for high-performance nutrition in chapters 3 through 5. Also include what *time* you eat each meal.

Breakfast _____

Snack _____

Lunch _____

Snack _____

Dinner _____

Snack _____

Daily fluid intake _____
(Aim for ½ to 1 ounce per pound of body weight. Example: if you weigh 160 pounds, you should drink between one and a half and three 1.5 liter bottles of water.)

Coffee, tea, sodas _____
(Always drink these in moderation since they contain caffeine and sugar. Most of your daily fluid intake should be water.)

High-Performance Nutrition Supplementation

No supplementation unless you make this your optional cardio day. In that case, follow the Wednesday supplementation schedule on page 108.

Daily Exercise

Remember, this routine is optional. Following the guidelines in chapters 8 through 11, check off the items that apply.

I performed my general warm-up and stretching routine at the proper RPE

_____

I performed my specific warm-up (stretches) at the proper RPE _____

I performed my pelvic stabilizer exercises in the order indicated ____

I completed all my sets and reps ____ Amount of weight used ____

I performed my cardiovascular exercise ____

I performed my cooldown routine at the proper RPE ____

I performed my second set of pelvic stabilizers in the order indicated ____

I performed all my sets and reps ____ (no weights required)

How I felt at the end of my workout _____

Week 2, Day 7

Rest and Recovery Day

High-Performance Nutrition

Use the guidelines for high-performance nutrition in chapters 3 through 5. Also include what *time* you eat each meal.

Breakfast _____

Snack _____

Lunch _____

Snack _____

Dinner _____

Snack _____

Daily fluid intake _____

(Aim for $\frac{1}{2}$ to 1 ounce per pound of body weight. Example: if you weigh 160 pounds, you should drink between one and a half and three 1.5 liter bottles of water.)

Coffee, tea, sodas _____

(Always drink these in moderation since they contain caffeine and sugar. Most of your daily fluid intake should be water.)

High-Performance Nutrition Supplementation

No supplementation.

No Exercise

Make this a true rest-and-recovery day. This practice will greatly enhance your body's energy and muscle-building capacity. See chapter 1 for the reasons behind taking rest-and-recovery days.

Week 3, Day 1

High-Performance Nutrition

Use the guidelines for high-performance nutrition in chapters 3 through 5. Also include what *time* you eat each meal.

Breakfast _____

Snack _____

Lunch _____

Snack _____

Dinner _____

Snack _____

Daily fluid intake _____
(Aim for ½ to 1 ounce per pound of body weight. Example: if you weigh 160 pounds, you should drink between one and a half and three 1.5 liter bottles of water.)

Coffee, tea, sodas _____
(Always drink these in moderation since they contain caffeine and sugar. Most of your daily fluid intake should be water.)

High-Performance Nutrition Supplementation

Following the guidelines in chapters 6 and 7, check off the items that apply.

I took my preworkout supplements _____

I stayed hydrated during my workout _____

I took my postworkout supplements _____

I took my presleep supplements _____

I took my multivitamins/minerals and antioxidants on schedule _____

Daily Exercise

Following the guidelines in chapters 8 through 11, check off the items that apply.

I performed my general warm-up and stretching routine at the proper RPE _____

I performed my specific warm-up at the proper RPE _____

I performed my energy system management exercises at the proper RPE _____

I allowed my heart rate (HR) to recover to 120 bpm _____

I performed my cooldown at the proper RPE _____

I did my upper body exercises in the order indicated ____

I completed all my sets and reps ____ Amount of weight used ____

I performed my pelvic stabilizers ____

I completed all my sets and reps ____ (no weights required)

How I felt at the end of my workout _____

Week 3, Day 2

High-Performance Nutrition

Use the guidelines for high-performance nutrition in chapters 3 through 5. Also include what *time* you eat each meal.

Breakfast _____

Snack _____

Lunch _____

Snack _____

Dinner _____

Snack _____

Daily fluid intake _____

(Aim for $\frac{1}{2}$ to 1 ounce per pound of body weight. Example: if you weigh 160 pounds, you should drink between one and a half and three 1.5 liter bottles of water.)

Coffee, tea, sodas _____

(Always drink these in moderation since they contain caffeine and sugar. Most of your daily fluid intake should be water.)

High-Performance Nutrition Supplementation

Following the guidelines in chapters 6 and 7, check off the items that apply.

I took my preworkout supplements ____

I stayed hydrated during my workout ____

I took my postworkout supplements ____

I took my presleep supplements ____

I took my multivitamins/minerals and antioxidants on schedule ____

Daily Exercise

Following the guidelines in chapters 8 through 11, check off the items that apply.

I performed my general warm-up and stretching routine at the proper RPE ____

I performed my pelvic stabilizer exercises in the order indicated ____

I performed my lower body exercises in the order indicated ____

I completed all my sets and reps ____ Amount of weight used ____

I performed my general warm-up at the proper RPE ____

I performed my specific warm-up at the proper RPE ____

I performed my energy system management exercises at the proper RPE ____

I allowed my HR to recover to 130 bpm ____

I performed my cooldown at the proper RPE ____

How I felt at the end of my workout _____

Week 3, Day 3

Optional Cardio Day

High-Performance Nutrition

Use the guidelines for high-performance nutrition in chapters 3 through 5. Also include what *time* you eat each meal.

Breakfast _____

Snack _____

Lunch _____

Snack _____

Dinner _____

Snack _____

Daily fluid intake _____
(Aim for ½ to 1 ounce per pound of body weight. Example: if you weigh 160 pounds, you should drink between one and a half and three 1.5 liter bottles of water.)

Coffee, tea, sodas _____
(Always drink these in moderation since they contain caffeine and sugar. Most of your daily fluid intake should be water.)

High-Performance Nutrition Supplementation

Following the guidelines in chapters 6 and 7, check off the items that apply.

I took my preworkout supplements ____

I stayed hydrated during my workout _____

I took my postworkout supplements _____

I took my presleep supplements

I took my multivitamins/minerals and antioxidants on schedule _____

If this is a nonworkout day, take no supplementation.

Daily Exercise

Remember, this routine is optional. Following the guidelines in chapters 8 through 11, check off the items that apply.

I performed my general warm-up and stretching routine at the proper RPE _____

I performed my specific warm-up (stretches) at the proper RPE _____

I performed my pelvic stabilizer exercises in the order indicated _____

I completed all my sets and reps _____ Amount of weight used _____

I performed my cardiovascular exercise _____

I performed my cooldown routine at the proper RPE _____

I performed my second set of pelvic stabilizers in the order indicated _____

I performed all my sets and reps _____ (no weights required)

How I felt at the end of my workout _____

Week 3, Day 4

High-Performance Nutrition

Use the guidelines for high-performance nutrition in chapters 3 through 5. Also include what *time* you eat each meal.

Breakfast _____

Snack _____

Lunch _____

Snack _____

Dinner _____

Snack _____

Daily fluid intake _____
(Aim for ½ to 1 ounce per pound of body weight. Example: if you weigh 160 pounds, you should drink between one and a half and three 1.5 liter bottles of water.)

Coffee, tea, sodas _____

(Always drink these in moderation since they contain caffeine and sugar. Most of your daily fluid intake should be water.)

High-Performance Nutrition Supplementation

Following the guidelines in chapters 6 and 7, check off the items that apply.

I took my preworkout supplements ____

I stayed hydrated during my workout ____

I took my postworkout supplements ____

I took my presleep supplements ____

I took my multivitamins/minerals and antioxidants on schedule ____

Daily Exercise

Following the guidelines in chapters 8 through 11, check off the items that apply.

I performed my general warm-up and stretching routine at the proper RPE ____

I performed my specific warm-up routine at the proper RPE ____

I performed my energy system management exercises at the proper RPE ____

I allowed my HR to recover to 120 bpm ____

I performed my cooldown at the proper RPE ____

I performed my upper body exercises in the order indicated ____

I completed all my sets and reps ____ Amount of weight used ____

I performed my pelvic stabilizers in the order indicated ____

I performed the required sets and repetitions (weights not used) ____

How I felt at the end of my workout _____

Week 3, Day 5

High-Performance Nutrition

Use the guidelines for high-performance nutrition in chapters 3 through 5. Also include what *time* you eat each meal.

Breakfast _____

Snack _____

Lunch _____

Snack _____

Dinner _____

Snack _____

Daily fluid intake _____
(Aim for ½ to 1 ounce per pound of body weight. Example: if you weigh 160 pounds, you should drink between one and a half and three 1.5 liter bottles of water.)

Coffee, tea, sodas _____
(Always drink these in moderation since they contain caffeine and sugar. Most of your daily fluid intake should be water.)

High-Performance Nutrition Supplementation

Following the guidelines in chapters 6 and 7, check off the items that apply.

I took my preworkout supplements _____

I stayed hydrated during my workout _____

I took my postworkout supplements _____

I took my presleep supplements _____

I took my multivitamins/minerals and antioxidants on schedule _____

Daily Exercise

Following the guidelines in chapters 8 through 11, check off the items that apply.

I performed my general warm-up and stretching routine at the proper RPE _____

I performed my pelvic stabilizer exercises in the order indicated _____

I performed my lower body exercises in the order indicated _____

I completed all my sets and reps _____ Amount of weight used _____

I performed my general warm-up at the proper RPE _____

I performed my specific warm-up at the proper RPE _____

I performed my energy system management exercises at the proper RPE _____

I allowed my HR to recover to 130 bpm _____

I performed my cooldown at the proper RPE _____

I stretched as needed _____

How I felt at the end of my workout _____

Week 3, Day 6

Optional Cardio Day

High-Performance Nutrition

Use the guidelines for high-performance nutrition in chapters 3 through 5. Also include what *time* you eat each meal.

Breakfast _____

Snack _____

Lunch _____

Snack _____

Dinner _____

Snack _____

Daily fluid intake _____
(Aim for ½ to 1 ounce per pound of body weight. Example: if you weigh 160 pounds, you should drink between one and a half and three 1.5 liter bottles of water.)

Coffee, tea, sodas _____
(Always drink these in moderation since they contain caffeine and sugar. Most of your daily fluid intake should be water.)

High-Performance Nutrition Supplementation

No supplementation unless you make this your optional cardio day. In that case, follow the Wednesday supplementation schedule on page 108.

Daily Exercise

Remember, this routine is optional. Following the guidelines in chapters 8 through 11, check off the items that apply.

I performed my general warm-up and stretching routine at the proper RPE ____

I performed my specific warm-up (stretches) at the proper RPE ____

I performed my pelvic stabilizer exercises in the order indicated ____

I completed all my sets and reps ____ Amount of weight used ____

I performed my cardiovascular exercise ____

I performed my cooldown routine at the proper RPE ____

I performed my second set of pelvic stabilizers in the order indicated ____

I performed all my sets and reps ____ (no weights required)

How I felt at the end of my workout _____

Week 3, Day 7

Rest and Recovery Day

High-Performance Nutrition

Use the guidelines for high-performance nutrition in chapters 3 through 5. Also include what *time* you eat each meal.

Breakfast _____

Snack _____

Lunch _____

Snack _____

Dinner _____

Snack _____

Daily fluid intake _____
(Aim for $\frac{1}{2}$ to 1 ounce per pound of body weight. Example: if you weigh 160 pounds, you should drink between one and a half and three 1.5 liter bottles of water.)

Coffee, tea, sodas _____
(Always drink these in moderation since they contain caffeine and sugar. Most of your daily fluid intake should be water.)

High-Performance Nutrition Supplementation

No supplementation.

No Exercise

Make this a true rest-and-recovery day. This practice will greatly enhance your body's energy and muscle-building capacity. See chapter 1 for the reasons behind taking rest-and-recovery days.

Week 4, Day 1

High-Performance Nutrition

Use the guidelines for high-performance nutrition in chapters 3 through 5. Also include what *time* you eat each meal.

Breakfast _____

Snack _____

Lunch _____

Snack _____

Dinner _____

Snack _____

Daily fluid intake _____

(Aim for ½ to 1 ounce per pound of body weight. Example: if you weigh 160 pounds, you should drink between one and a half and three 1.5 liter bottles of water.)

Coffee, tea, sodas _____

(Always drink these in moderation since they contain caffeine and sugar. Most of your daily fluid intake should be water.)

High-Performance Nutrition Supplementation

Following the guidelines in chapters 6 and 7, check off the items that apply.

I took my preworkout supplements ____

I stayed hydrated during my workout ____

I took my postworkout supplements ____

I took my presleep supplements ____

I took my multivitamins/minerals and antioxidants on schedule ____

Daily Exercise

Following the guidelines in chapters 8 through 11, check off the items that apply.

I performed my general warm-up and stretching routine at the proper RPE ____

I performed my specific warm-up at the proper RPE ____

I performed my energy system management exercises at the proper RPE ____

I allowed my heart rate (HR) to recover to 120 bpm ____

I performed my cooldown at the proper RPE ____

I did my upper body exercises in the order indicated ____

I completed all my sets and reps ____ Amount of weight used ____

I performed my pelvic stabilizers ____

I completed all my sets and reps ____ (no weights required)

How I felt at the end of my workout _____

Week 4, Day 2

High-Performance Nutrition

Use the guidelines for high-performance nutrition in chapters 3 through 5. Also include what *time* you eat each meal.

Breakfast _____

Snack _____

Lunch _____

Snack _____

Dinner _____

Snack _____

Daily fluid intake _____
(Aim for ½ to 1 ounce per pound of body weight. Example: if you weigh 160 pounds, you should drink between one and a half and three 1.5 liter bottles of water.)

Coffee, tea, sodas _____
(Always drink these in moderation since they contain caffeine and sugar. Most of your daily fluid intake should be water.)

High-Performance Nutrition Supplementation

Following the guidelines in chapters 6 and 7, check off the items that apply.

I took my preworkout supplements _____

I stayed hydrated during my workout _____

I took my postworkout supplements _____

I took my presleep supplements _____

I took my multivitamins/minerals and antioxidants on schedule _____

Daily Exercise

Following the guidelines in chapters 8 through 11, check off the items that apply.

I performed my general warm-up and stretching routine at the proper RPE _____

I performed my pelvic stabilizer exercises in the order indicated _____

I performed my lower body exercises in the order indicated _____

I completed all my sets and reps _____ Amount of weight used _____

I performed my general warm-up at the proper RPE _____

I performed my specific warm-up at the proper RPE _____

I performed my energy system management exercises at the proper RPE _____

I allowed my HR to recover to 130 bpm _____

I performed my cooldown at the proper RPE _____

How I felt at the end of my workout _____

Week 4, Day 3

Optional Cardio Day

High-Performance Nutrition

Use the guidelines for high-performance nutrition in chapters 3 through 5. Also include what *time* you eat each meal.

Breakfast _____

Snack _____

Lunch _____

Snack _____

Dinner _____

Snack _____

Daily fluid intake _____
(Aim for ½ to 1 ounce per pound of body weight. Example: if you weigh 160 pounds, you should drink between one and a half and three 1.5 liter bottles of water.)

Coffee, tea, sodas _____
(Always drink these in moderation since they contain caffeine and sugar. Most of your daily fluid intake should be water.)

High-Performance Nutrition Supplementation

Following the guidelines in chapters 6 and 7, check off the items that apply.

I took my preworkout supplements _____

I stayed hydrated during my workout _____

I took my postworkout supplements _____

I took my presleep supplements

I took my multivitamins/minerals and antioxidants on schedule _____

If this is a nonworkout day, take no supplementation.

Daily Exercise

Remember, this routine is optional. Following the guidelines in chapters 8 through 11, check off the items that apply.

I performed my general warm-up and stretching routine at the proper RPE _____

I performed my specific warm-up (stretches) at the proper RPE _____

I performed my pelvic stabilizer exercises in the order indicated _____

I completed all my sets and reps _____ Amount of weight used _____

I performed my cardiovascular exercise _____

I performed my cooldown routine at the proper RPE _____

I performed my second set of pelvic stabilizers in the order indicated _____

I performed all my sets and reps _____ (no weights required)

How I felt at the end of my workout _____

Week 4, Day 4

High-Performance Nutrition

Use the guidelines for high-performance nutrition in chapters 3 through 5. Also include what *time* you eat each meal.

Breakfast _____

Snack _____

Lunch _____

Snack _____

Dinner _____

Snack _____

Daily fluid intake _____
(Aim for ½ to 1 ounce per pound of body weight. Example: if you weigh 160 pounds, you should drink between one and a half and three 1.5 liter bottles of water.)

Coffee, tea, sodas _____
(Always drink these in moderation since they contain caffeine and sugar. Most of your daily fluid intake should be water.)

High-Performance Nutrition Supplementation

Following the guidelines in chapters 6 and 7, check off the items that apply.

I took my preworkout supplements _____

I stayed hydrated during my workout _____

I took my postworkout supplements _____

I took my presleep supplements _____

I took my multivitamins/minerals and antioxidants on schedule _____

Daily Exercise

Following the guidelines in chapters 8 through 11, check off the items that apply.

I performed my general warm-up and stretching routine at the proper RPE
____

I performed my specific warm-up routine at the proper RPE ____

I performed my energy system management exercises at the proper RPE ____

I allowed my HR to recover to 120 bpm ____

I performed my cooldown at the proper RPE ____

I performed my upper body exercises in the order indicated ____

I completed all my sets and reps ____ Amount of weight used ____

I performed my pelvic stabilizers in the order indicated ____

I performed the required sets and repetitions (weights not used) ____

How I felt at the end of my workout _____

Week 4, Day 5

High-Performance Nutrition

Use the guidelines for high-performance nutrition in chapters 3 through 5. Also include what *time* you eat each meal.

Breakfast _____

Snack _____

Lunch _____

Snack _____

Dinner _____

Snack _____

Daily fluid intake _____
(Aim for ½ to 1 ounce per pound of body weight. Example: if you weigh 160 pounds, you should drink between one and a half and three 1.5 liter bottles of water.)

Coffee, tea, sodas _____
(Always drink these in moderation since they contain caffeine and sugar. Most of your daily fluid intake should be water.)

High-Performance Nutrition Supplementation

Following the guidelines in chapters 6 and 7, check off the items that apply.

I took my preworkout supplements ____

I stayed hydrated during my workout ____

I took my postworkout supplements ____

I took my presleep supplements ____

I took my multivitamins/minerals and antioxidants on schedule ____

Daily Exercise

Following the guidelines in chapters 8 through 11, check off the items that apply.

I performed my general warm-up and stretching routine at the proper RPE ____

I performed my pelvic stabilizer exercises in the order indicated ____

I performed my lower body exercises in the order indicated ____

I completed all my sets and reps ____ Amount of weight used ____

I performed my general warm-up at the proper RPE ____

I performed my specific warm-up at the proper RPE ____

I performed my energy system management exercises at the proper RPE ____

I allowed my HR to recover to 130 bpm ____

I performed my cooldown at the proper RPE ____

I stretched as needed ____

How I felt at the end of my workout _____

Week 4, Day 6

Optional Cardio Day

High-Performance Nutrition

Use the guidelines for high-performance nutrition in chapters 3 through 5. Also include what *time* you eat each meal.

Breakfast _____

Snack _____

Lunch _____

Snack _____

Dinner _____

Snack _____

Daily fluid intake _____
(Aim for ½ to 1 ounce per pound of body weight. Example: if you weigh 160 pounds, you should drink between one and a half and three 1.5 liter bottles of water.)

Coffee, tea, sodas _____

(Always drink these in moderation since they contain caffeine and sugar. Most of your daily fluid intake should be water.)

High-Performance Nutrition Supplementation

No supplementation unless you make this your optional cardio day. In that case, follow the Wednesday supplementation schedule on page 108.

Daily Exercise

Remember, this routine is optional. Following the guidelines in chapters 8 through 11, check off the items that apply.

I performed my general warm-up and stretching routine at the proper RPE

_____

I performed my specific warm-up (stretches) at the proper RPE ____

I performed my pelvic stabilizer exercises in the order indicated ____

I completed all my sets and reps ____ Amount of weight used ____

I performed my cardiovascular exercise ____

I performed my cooldown routine at the proper RPE ____

I performed my second set of pelvic stabilizers in the order indicated ____

I performed all my sets and reps ____ (no weights required)

How I felt at the end of my workout _____

Week 4, Day 7

Rest and Recovery Day

High-Performance Nutrition

Use the guidelines for high-performance nutrition in chapters 3 through 5. Also include what *time* you eat each meal.

Breakfast _____

Snack _____

Lunch _____

Snack _____

Dinner _____

Snack _____

Daily fluid intake _____

(Aim for ½ to 1 ounce per pound of body weight. Example: if you weigh 160 pounds, you should drink between one and a half and three 1.5 liter bottles of water.)

Coffee, tea, sodas _____
(Always drink these in moderation since they contain caffeine and sugar. Most of your daily fluid intake should be water.)

High-Performance Nutrition Supplementation

No supplementation.

No Exercise

Make this a true rest-and-recovery day. This practice will greatly enhance your body's energy and muscle-building capacity. See chapter 1 for the reasons behind taking rest-and-recovery days.

Week 5, Day 1

High-Performance Nutrition

Use the guidelines for high-performance nutrition in chapters 3 through 5. Also include what *time* you eat each meal.

Breakfast _____

Snack _____

Lunch _____

Snack _____

Dinner _____

Snack _____

Daily fluid intake _____
(Aim for ½ to 1 ounce per pound of body weight. Example: if you weigh 160 pounds, you should drink between one and a half and three 1.5 liter bottles of water.)

Coffee, tea, sodas _____
(Always drink these in moderation since they contain caffeine and sugar. Most of your daily fluid intake should be water.)

High-Performance Nutrition Supplementation

Following the guidelines in chapters 6 and 7, check off the items that apply.

I took my preworkout supplements _____

I stayed hydrated during my workout _____

I took my postworkout supplements _____

I took my presleep supplements _____

I took my multivitamins/minerals and antioxidants on schedule _____

Daily Exercise

Following the guidelines in chapters 8 through 11, check off the items that apply.

I performed my general warm-up and stretching routine at the proper RPE

_____

I performed my specific warm-up at the proper RPE _____

I performed my energy system management exercises at the proper RPE _____

I allowed my heart rate (HR) to recover to 120 bpm _____

I performed my cooldown at the proper RPE _____

I did my upper body exercises in the order indicated _____

I completed all my sets and reps _____ Amount of weight used _____

I performed my pelvic stabilizers _____

I completed all my sets and reps _____ (no weights required)

How I felt at the end of my workout _____

Week 5, Day 2

High-Performance Nutrition

Use the guidelines for high-performance nutrition in chapters 3 through 5. Also include what *time* you eat each meal.

Breakfast _____

Snack _____

Lunch _____

Snack _____

Dinner _____

Snack _____

Daily fluid intake _____
(Aim for ½ to 1 ounce per pound of body weight. Example: if you weigh 160 pounds, you should drink between one and a half and three 1.5 liter bottles of water.)

Coffee, tea, sodas _____
(Always drink these in moderation since they contain caffeine and sugar. Most of your daily fluid intake should be water.)

High-Performance Nutrition Supplementation

Following the guidelines in chapters 6 and 7, check off the items that apply.

I took my preworkout supplements ____

I stayed hydrated during my workout ____

I took my postworkout supplements ____

I took my presleep supplements ____

I took my multivitamins/minerals and antioxidants on schedule ____

Daily Exercise

Following the guidelines in chapters 8 through 11, check off the items that apply.

I performed my general warm-up and stretching routine at the proper RPE ____

I performed my pelvic stabilizer exercises in the order indicated ____

I performed my lower body exercises in the order indicated ____

I completed all my sets and reps ____ Amount of weight used ____

I performed my general warm-up at the proper RPE ____

I performed my specific warm-up at the proper RPE ____

I performed my energy system management exercises at the proper RPE ____

I allowed my HR to recover to 120 bpm ____

I performed my cooldown at the proper RPE ____

How I felt at the end of my workout _____

Week 5, Day 3

Optional Cardio Day

High-Performance Nutrition

Use the guidelines for high-performance nutrition in chapters 3 through 5. Also include what *time* you eat each meal.

Breakfast _____

Snack _____

Lunch _____

Snack _____

Dinner _____

Snack _____

Daily fluid intake _____
(Aim for ½ to 1 ounce per pound of body weight. Example: if you weigh 160 pounds, you should drink between one and a half and three 1.5 liter bottles of water.)

Coffee, tea, sodas _____
(Always drink these in moderation since they contain caffeine and sugar. Most of your daily fluid intake should be water.)

High-Performance Nutrition Supplementation

Following the guidelines in chapters 6 and 7, check off the items that apply.

I took my preworkout supplements ____

I stayed hydrated during my workout ____

I took my postworkout supplements ____

I took my multivitamins/minerals and antioxidants on schedule ____

If this is a nonworkout day, take no supplementation.

Daily Exercise

Remember, this routine is optional. Following the guidelines in chapters 8 through 11, check off the items that apply.

I performed my general warm-up and stretching routine at the proper RPE ____

I performed my specific warm-up (stretches) at the proper RPE ____

I performed my pelvic stabilizer exercises in the order indicated ____

I completed all my sets and reps ____ Amount of weight used ____

I performed my cardiovascular exercise ____

I performed my cooldown routine at the proper RPE ____

I performed my second set of pelvic stabilizers in the order indicated ____

I performed all my sets and reps ____ (no weights required)

How I felt at the end of my workout _____

Week 5, Day 4

High-Performance Nutrition

Use the guidelines for high-performance nutrition in chapters 3 through 5. Also include what *time* you eat each meal.

Breakfast _____

Snack _____

Lunch _____

Snack _____

Dinner _____

Snack _____

Daily fluid intake _____
(Aim for ½ to 1 ounce per pound of body weight. Example: if you weigh 160 pounds, you should drink between one and a half and three 1.5 liter bottles of water.)

Coffee, tea, sodas _____
(Always drink these in moderation since they contain caffeine and sugar. Most of your daily fluid intake should be water.)

High-Performance Nutrition Supplementation

Following the guidelines in chapters 6 and 7, check off the items that apply.

I took my preworkout supplements _____

I stayed hydrated during my workout _____

I took my postworkout supplements _____

I took my presleep supplements _____

I took my multivitamins/minerals and antioxidants on schedule _____

Daily Exercise

Following the guidelines in chapters 8 through 11, check off the items that apply.

I performed my general warm-up and stretching routine at the proper RPE _____

I performed my specific warm-up routine at the proper RPE _____

I performed my energy system management exercises at the proper RPE _____

I allowed my HR to recover to 120 bpm _____

I performed my cooldown at the proper RPE _____

I performed my upper body exercises in the order indicated _____

I completed all my sets and reps _____ Amount of weight used _____

I performed my pelvic stabilizers in the order indicated _____

I performed the required sets and repetitions (weights not used) _____

How I felt at the end of my workout _____

Week 5, Day 5

High-Performance Nutrition

Use the guidelines for high-performance nutrition in chapters 3 through 5. Also include what *time* you eat each meal.

Breakfast _____

Snack _____

Lunch _____

Snack _____

Dinner _____

Snack _____

Daily fluid intake _____
(Aim for ½ to 1 ounce per pound of body weight. Example: if you weigh 160 pounds, you should drink between one and a half and three 1.5 liter bottles of water.)

Coffee, tea, sodas _____
(Always drink these in moderation since they contain caffeine and sugar. Most of your daily fluid intake should be water.)

High-Performance Nutrition Supplementation

Following the guidelines in chapters 6 and 7, check off the items that apply.

I took my preworkout supplements _____

I stayed hydrated during my workout _____

I took my postworkout supplements _____

I took my presleep supplements _____

I took my multivitamins/minerals and antioxidants on schedule _____

Daily Exercise

Following the guidelines in chapters 8 through 11, check off the items that apply.

I performed my general warm-up and stretching routine at the proper RPE _____

I performed my specific warm-up routine at the proper RPE _____

I performed my energy system management exercises at the proper RPE _____

I allowed my HR to recover to 120 bpm _____

I performed my cooldown at the proper RPE _____

I performed my upper body exercises in the order indicated ____

I completed all my sets and reps ____ Amount of weight used ____

I performed my pelvic stabilizers in the order indicated ____

I performed the required sets and repetitions (weights not used) ____

How I felt at the end of my workout _____

Week 5, Day 6

Optional Cardio Day

High-Performance Nutrition

Use the guidelines for high-performance nutrition in chapters 3 through 5. Also include what *time* you eat each meal.

Breakfast _____

Snack _____

Lunch _____

Snack _____

Dinner _____

Snack _____

Daily fluid intake _____
(Aim for ½ to 1 ounce per pound of body weight. Example: if you weigh 160 pounds, you should drink between one and a half and three 1.5 liter bottles of water.)

Coffee, tea, sodas _____
(Always drink these in moderation since they contain caffeine and sugar. Most of your daily fluid intake should be water.)

High-Performance Nutrition Supplementation

No supplementation unless you make this your optional cardio day. In that case, follow the Wednesday supplementation schedule on page 109.

Daily Exercise

Remember, this routine is optional. Following the guidelines in chapters 8 through 11, check off the items that apply.

I performed my general warm-up and stretching routine at the proper RPE ____

I performed my specific warm-up (stretches) at the proper RPE ____

I performed my pelvic stabilizer exercises in the order indicated _____

I completed all my sets and reps _____ Amount of weight used _____

I performed my cardiovascular exercise _____

I performed my cooldown routine at the proper RPE _____

I performed my second set of pelvic stabilizers in the order indicated _____

I performed all my sets and reps _____ (no weights required)

How I felt at the end of my workout _____

Week 5, Day 7

Rest and Recovery Day

High-Performance Nutrition

Use the guidelines for high-performance nutrition in chapters 3 through 5. Also include what *time* you eat each meal.

Breakfast _____

Snack _____

Lunch _____

Snack _____

Dinner _____

Snack _____

Daily fluid intake _____

(Aim for ½ to 1 ounce per pound of body weight. Example: if you weigh 160 pounds, you should drink between one and a half and three 1.5 liter bottles of water.)

Coffee, tea, sodas _____

(Always drink these in moderation since they contain caffeine and sugar. Most of your daily fluid intake should be water.)

High-Performance Nutrition Supplementation

No supplementation.

No Exercise

Make this a true rest-and-recovery day. This practice will greatly enhance your body's energy and muscle-building capacity. See chapter 1 for the reasons behind taking rest-and-recovery days.

Week 6, Day 1

High-Performance Nutrition

Use the guidelines for high-performance nutrition in chapters 3 through 5. Also include what *time* you eat each meal.

Breakfast _____

Snack _____

Lunch _____

Snack _____

Dinner _____

Snack _____

Daily fluid intake _____
(Aim for ½ to 1 ounce per pound of body weight. Example: if you weigh 160 pounds, you should drink between one and a half and three 1.5 liter bottles of water.)

Coffee, tea, sodas _____
(Always drink these in moderation since they contain caffeine and sugar. Most of your daily fluid intake should be water.)

High-Performance Nutrition Supplementation

Following the guidelines in chapters 6 and 7, check off the items that apply.

I took my preworkout supplements _____

I stayed hydrated during my workout _____

I took my postworkout supplements _____

I took my multivitamins/minerals and antioxidants on schedule _____

Daily Exercise

Following the guidelines in chapters 8 through 11, check off the items that apply.

I performed my general warm-up and stretching routine at the proper RPE _____

I performed my specific warm-up at the proper RPE _____

I performed my energy system management exercises at the proper RPE _____

I allowed my heart rate (HR) to recover to 120 bpm _____

I performed my cooldown at the proper RPE _____

I did my upper body exercises in the order indicated _____

I completed all my sets and reps _____ Amount of weight used _____

I performed my pelvic stabilizers _____

I completed all my sets and reps _____ (no weights required)

How I felt at the end of my workout _____

Week 6, Day 2

High-Performance Nutrition

Use the guidelines for high-performance nutrition in chapters 3 through 5. Also include what *time* you eat each meal.

Breakfast _____

Snack _____

Lunch _____

Snack _____

Dinner _____

Snack _____

Daily fluid intake _____
(Aim for ½ to 1 ounce per pound of body weight. Example: if you weigh 160 pounds, you should drink between one and a half and three 1.5 liter bottles of water.)

Coffee, tea, sodas _____
(Always drink these in moderation since they contain caffeine and sugar. Most of your daily fluid intake should be water.)

High-Performance Nutrition Supplementation

Following the guidelines in chapters 6 and 7, check off the items that apply.

I took my preworkout supplements _____

I stayed hydrated during my workout _____

I took my postworkout supplements _____

I took my multivitamins/minerals and antioxidants on schedule _____

Daily Exercise

Following the guidelines in chapters 8 through 11, check off the items that apply.

I performed my general warm-up and stretching routine at the proper RPE _____

I performed my pelvic stabilizer exercises in the order indicated ____

I performed my lower body exercises in the order indicated ____

I completed all my sets and reps ____ Amount of weight used ____

I performed my general warm-up at the proper RPE ____

I performed my specific warm-up at the proper RPE ____

I performed my energy system management exercises at the proper RPE ____

I allowed my HR to recover to 130 bpm ____

I performed my cooldown at the proper RPE ____

How I felt at the end of my workout _____

Week 6, Day 3

Optional Cardio Day

High-Performance Nutrition

Use the guidelines for high-performance nutrition in chapters 3 through 5. Also include what *time* you eat each meal.

Breakfast _____

Snack _____

Lunch _____

Snack _____

Dinner _____

Snack _____

Daily fluid intake _____
(Aim for ½ to 1 ounce per pound of body weight. Example: if you weigh 160 pounds, you should drink between one and a half and three 1.5 liter bottles of water.)

Coffee, tea, sodas _____
(Always drink these in moderation since they contain caffeine and sugar. Most of your daily fluid intake should be water.)

High-Performance Nutrition Supplementation

Following the guidelines in chapters 6 and 7, check off the items that apply.

I took my preworkout supplements ____

I stayed hydrated during my workout ____

I took my postworkout supplements ____

I took my presleep supplements ____

I took my multivitamins/minerals and antioxidants on schedule ____

If this is a nonworkout day, take no supplementation.

Daily Exercise

Remember, this routine is optional. Following the guidelines in chapters 8 through 11, check off the items that apply.

I performed my general warm-up and stretching routine at the proper RPE

____

I performed my specific warm-up (stretches) at the proper RPE ____

I performed my pelvic stabilizer exercises in the order indicated ____

I completed all my sets and reps ____ Amount of weight used ____

I performed my cardiovascular exercise ____

I performed my cooldown routine at the proper RPE ____

I performed my second set of pelvic stabilizers in the order indicated ____

I performed all my sets and reps ____ (no weights required)

How I felt at the end of my workout _____

Week 6, Day 4

High-Performance Nutrition

Use the guidelines for high-performance nutrition in chapters 3 through 5. Also include what *time* you eat each meal.

Breakfast _____

Snack _____

Lunch _____

Snack _____

Dinner _____

Snack _____

Daily fluid intake _____

(Aim for ½ to 1 ounce per pound of body weight. Example: if you weigh 160 pounds, you should drink between one and a half and three 1.5 liter bottles of water.)

Coffee, tea, sodas _____

(Always drink these in moderation since they contain caffeine and sugar. Most of your daily fluid intake should be water.)

High-Performance Nutrition Supplementation
Following the guidelines in chapters 6 and 7, check off the items that apply.

I took my preworkout supplements _____

I stayed hydrated during my workout _____

I took my postworkout supplements _____

I took my presleep supplements _____

I took my multivitamins/minerals and antioxidants on schedule _____

Daily Exercise
Following the guidelines in chapters 8 through 11, check off the items that apply.

I performed my general warm-up and stretching routine at the proper RPE _____

I performed my specific warm-up routine at the proper RPE _____

I performed my energy system management exercises at the proper RPE _____

I allowed my HR to recover to 120 bpm _____

I performed my cooldown at the proper RPE _____

I performed my upper body exercises in the order indicated _____

I completed all my sets and reps _____ Amount of weight used _____

I performed my pelvic stabilizers in the order indicated _____

I performed the required sets and repetitions (weights not used) _____

How I felt at the end of my workout _____

Week 6, Day 5

High-Performance Nutrition
Use the guidelines for high-performance nutrition in chapters 3 through 5. Also include what *time* you eat each meal.

Breakfast _____

Snack _____

Lunch _____

Snack _____

Dinner _____

Snack _____

Daily fluid intake _____
(Aim for ½ to 1 ounce per pound of body weight. Example: if you weigh 160 pounds, you should drink between one and a half and three 1.5 liter bottles of water.)

Coffee, tea, sodas _____
(Always drink these in moderation since they contain caffeine and sugar. Most of your daily fluid intake should be water.)

High-Performance Nutrition Supplementation

Following the guidelines in chapters 6 and 7, check off the items that apply.

I took my preworkout supplements ____

I stayed hydrated during my workout ____

I took my postworkout supplements ____

I took my multivitamins/minerals and antioxidants on schedule ____

Daily Exercise

Following the guidelines in chapters 8 through 11, check off the items that apply.

I performed my general warm-up and stretching routine at the proper RPE

____

I performed my pelvic stabilizer exercises in the order indicated ____

I performed my lower body exercises in the order indicated ____

I completed all my sets and reps ____ Amount of weight used ____

I performed my general warm-up at the proper RPE ____

I performed my specific warm-up at the proper RPE ____

I performed my energy system management exercises at the proper RPE

____

I allowed my HR to recover to 130 bpm ____

I performed my cooldown at the proper RPE ____

I stretched as needed ____

How I felt at the end of my workout _____

Week 6, Day 6

High-Performance Nutrition

Use the guidelines for high-performance nutrition in chapters 3 through 5. Also include what *time* you eat each meal.

Breakfast _____

Snack _____

Lunch _____

Snack _____

Dinner _____

Snack _____

Daily fluid intake _____
(Aim for ½ to 1 ounce per pound of body weight. Example: if you weigh 160 pounds, you should drink between one and a half and three 1.5 liter bottles of water.)

Coffee, tea, sodas _____
(Always drink these in moderation since they contain caffeine and sugar. Most of your daily fluid intake should be water.)

High-Performance Nutrition Supplementation

No supplementation unless you make this your optional cardio day. In that case, follow the Wednesday supplementation schedule on page 110.

Daily Exercise

Remember, this routine is optional. Following the guidelines in chapters 8 through 11, check off the items that apply.

I performed my general warm-up and stretching routine at the proper RPE ____

I performed my specific warm-up (stretches) at the proper RPE ____

I performed my pelvic stabilizer exercises in the order indicated ____

I completed all my sets and reps ____ Amount of weight used ____

I performed my cardiovascular exercise ____

I performed my cooldown routine at the proper RPE ____

I performed my second set of pelvic stabilizers in the order indicated ____

I performed all my sets and reps ____ (no weights required)

How I felt at the end of my workout _____

Week 6, Day 7

Rest and Recovery Day

High-Performance Nutrition

Use the guidelines for high-performance nutrition in chapters 3 through 5. Also include what *time* you eat each meal.

Breakfast _____

Snack _____

Lunch _____

Snack _____

Dinner _____

Snack _____

Daily fluid intake _____
(Aim for ½ to 1 ounce per pound of body weight. Example: if you weigh 160 pounds, you should drink between one and a half and three 1.5 liter bottles of water.)

Coffee, tea, sodas _____
(Always drink these in moderation since they contain caffeine and sugar. Most of your daily fluid intake should be water.)

High-Performance Nutrition Supplementation

No supplementation.

No Exercise

Make this a true rest-and-recovery day. This practice will greatly enhance your body's energy and muscle-building capacity. See chapter 1 for the reasons behind taking rest-and recovery-days.

Maintenance Schedule

To help you to keep your Lean and Hard Program muscle gains, I have designed a maintenance schedule of exercise and supplementation. Since you are no longer striving to gain muscle quickly, but to keep what you have—and even increase muscle, but at a slower rate—you will also be adjusting your daily caloric intake downward somewhat. Please see chapter 5 for a formula that will enable you to calculate your new number of daily calories ingested.

At a future date if you wish to return to the Lean and Hard six-week program for additional rapid muscle gains, you may do so.

Maintenance Program

Day 1

High-Performance Nutrition

Use the guidelines for high-performance nutrition in chapters 3 through 5. Also include what *time* you eat each meal.

Breakfast _____

Snack _____

Lunch _____

Snack _____

Dinner _____

Snack _____

Daily fluid intake _____
(Aim for ½ to 1 ounce per pound of body weight. Example: if you weigh 160 pounds, you should drink between one and a half and three 1.5 liter bottles of water.)

Coffee, tea, sodas _____
(Always drink these in moderation since they contain caffeine and sugar. Most of your daily fluid intake should be water.)

High-Performance Nutrition Supplementation

Following the guidelines in chapters 6 and 7, check off the items that apply.

I stayed hydrated using my favorite sports drink during my workout ____

I took my postworkout supplements ____

If my workout was longer than 45 minutes, I mixed my creatine monohydrate in juice for extra carbohydrate ____

I took my presleep supplementation ____

I only took my presleep maltodextrin if I worked out two consecutive days in a row ____

I took my multivitamins/minerals and antioxidants on schedule ____

Daily Exercise

Following the guidelines in chapters 8 through 11, check off the items that apply.

I performed my general warm-up and stretching routine at the proper RPE

____

I performed my specific warm-up at the proper RPE ____

I performed my energy system management exercises at the proper RPE ____

I allowed my HR to recover to 120 bpm ____

I performed my cooldown at the proper RPE ____

I did my upper body exercises in the order indicated ____

I completed all my sets and reps ____ Amount of weight used ____

I performed my pelvic stabilizer exercises ____

I completed all my sets and reps ____ (no weights required)

How I felt at the end of my workout _____

Day 2

High-Performance Nutrition

Use the guidelines for high-performance nutrition in chapters 3 through 5. Also include what *time* you eat each meal.

Breakfast _____

Snack _____

Lunch _____

Snack _____

Dinner _____

Snack _____

Daily fluid intake _____
(Aim for $\frac{1}{2}$ to 1 ounce per pound of body weight. Example: if you weigh 160 pounds, you should drink between one and a half and three 1.5 liter bottles of water.)

Coffee, tea, sodas _____
(Always drink these in moderation since they contain caffeine and sugar. Most of your daily fluid intake should be water.)

High-Performance Nutrition Supplementation

Following the guidelines in chapters 6 and 7, check off the items that apply.

I stayed hydrated using my favorite sports drink during my workout ____

I took my postworkout supplements ____

If my workout was longer than 45 minutes, I mixed my creatine monohydrate in juice for extra carbohydrate ____

I took my presleep supplementation ____

I only took my presleep maltodextrin if I worked out two consecutive days in a row _____

I took my multivitamins/minerals and antioxidants on schedule _____

Daily Exercise

Following the guidelines in chapters 8 through 11, check off the items that apply.

I performed my general warm-up and stretching routine at the proper RPE _____

I performed my pelvic stabilizer exercises in the order indicated _____

I performed my lower body exercises in the order indicated _____

I completed all my sets and reps _____ Amount of weight used _____

I performed my general warm-up at the proper RPE _____

I performed my specific warm-up at the proper RPE _____

I performed my energy system management exercises at the proper RPE _____

I allowed my HR to recover to 130 bpm _____

I performed my cooldown at the proper RPE _____

How I felt at the end of my workout _____

Day 3

Optional Cardio Day

High-Performance Nutrition

Use the guidelines for high-performance nutrition in chapters 3 through 5. Also include what *time* you eat each meal.

Breakfast _____

Snack _____

Lunch _____

Snack _____

Dinner _____

Snack _____

Daily fluid intake _____
(Aim for ½ to 1 ounce per pound of body weight. Example: if you weigh 160 pounds, you should drink between one and a half and three 1.5 liter bottles of water.)

Coffee, tea, sodas _____

(Always drink these in moderation since they contain caffeine and sugar. Most of your daily fluid intake should be water.)

High-Performance Nutrition Supplementation

Following the guidelines in chapters 6 and 7, check off the items that apply.

I stayed hydrated using my favorite sports drink during my workout ____

I took my postworkout supplements ____

If my workout was longer than 45 minutes, I mixed my creatine monohydrate in juice for extra carbohydrate ____

I took my presleep supplementation ____

I only took my presleep maltodextrin if I worked out two consecutive days in a row ____

I took my multivitamins/minerals and antioxidants on schedule ____

Daily Exercise

Remember, this routine is optional. Following the guidelines in chapters 8 through 11, check off the items that apply.

I performed my general warm-up and stretching routine at the proper RPE

____

I performed my specific warm-up (stretches) at the proper RPE ____

I performed my pelvic stabilizer exercises in the order indicated ____

I completed all my sets and reps ____ Amount of weight used ____

I performed my cardiovascular exercise ____

I performed my cooldown routine at the proper RPE ____

I performed my second set of pelvic stabilizer exercises in the order indicated

____

I performed all my sets and reps ____ (no weights required)

How I felt at the end of my workout _____

Day 4

High-Performance Nutrition

Use the guidelines for high-performance nutrition in chapters 3 through 5. Also include what *time* you eat each meal.

Breakfast _____

Snack _____

Lunch _____

Snack _____

Dinner _____

Snack _____

Daily fluid intake _____
(Aim for ½ to 1 ounce per pound of body weight. Example: if you weigh 160 pounds, you should drink between one and a half and three 1.5 liter bottles of water.)

Coffee, tea, sodas _____
(Always drink these in moderation since they contain caffeine and sugar. Most of your daily fluid intake should be water.)

High-Performance Nutrition Supplementation

Following the guidelines in chapters 6 and 7, check off the items that apply.

I stayed hydrated using my favorite sports drink during my workout _____

I took my postworkout supplements _____

If my workout was longer than 45 minutes, I mixed my creatine monohydrate in juice for extra carbohydrate _____

I took my presleep supplementation _____

I only took my presleep maltodextrin if I worked out two consecutive days in a row _____

I took my multivitamins/minerals and antioxidants on schedule _____

Daily Exercise

Following the guidelines in chapters 8 through 11, check off the items that apply.

I performed my general warm-up and stretching routine at the proper RPE _____

I performed my upper body exercises in the order indicated _____

I completed all my sets and reps _____ Amount of weight used _____

I performed my pelvic stabilizer exercises in the order indicated _____

I performed the required sets and reps (weights not used) _____

I performed my lower body exercises in the order indicated _____

I completed all my sets and reps _____ Amount of weight used _____

I performed my cooldown _____

How I felt at the end of my workout _____

Day 5

High-Performance Nutrition

Use the guidelines for high-performance nutrition in chapters 3 through 5. Also include what *time* you eat each meal.

Breakfast _____

Snack _____

Lunch _____

Snack _____

Dinner _____

Snack _____

Daily fluid intake _____
(Aim for ½ to 1 ounce per pound of body weight. Example: if you weigh 160 pounds, you should drink between one and a half and three 1.5 liter bottles of water.)

Coffee, tea, sodas _____
(Always drink these in moderation since they contain caffeine and sugar. Most of your daily fluid intake should be water.)

High-Performance Nutrition Supplementation

Following the guidelines in chapters 6 and 7, check off the items that apply.

I stayed hydrated using my favorite sports drink during my workout _____

I took my postworkout supplements _____

If my workout was longer than 45 minutes, I mixed my creatine monohydrate in juice for extra carbohydrate _____

I took my presleep supplementation _____

I only took my presleep maltodextrin if I worked out two consecutive days in a row _____

I took my multivitamins/minerals and antioxidants on schedule _____

Daily Exercise

Following the guidelines in chapters 8 through 11, check off the items that apply.

I performed my general warm-up and stretching routine at the proper RPE ____

I performed my specific warm-up at the proper RPE ____

I performed my energy system management exercises at the proper RPE ____ (note: half-gasser has been added to routine)

I allowed my HR to recover to 130 bpm ____

I performed my cooldown at the proper RPE ____

How I felt at the end of my workout _____

Day 6

Optional Cardio Day

High-Performance Nutrition

Use the guidelines for high-performance nutrition in chapters 3 through 5. Also include what *time* you eat each meal.

Breakfast _____

Snack _____

Lunch _____

Snack _____

Dinner _____

Snack _____

Daily fluid intake _____
(Aim for ½ to 1 ounce per pound of body weight. Example: if you weigh 160 pounds, you should drink between one and a half and three 1.5 liter bottles of water.)

Coffee, tea, sodas _____
(Always drink these in moderation since they contain caffeine and sugar. Most of your daily fluid intake should be water.)

High-Performance Nutrition Supplementation

Following the guidelines in chapters 6 and 7, check off the items that apply.

I took my preworkout supplements ____

I stayed hydrated during my workout ____

I took my postworkout supplements ____

I took my multivitamins/minerals and antioxidants on schedule ____

Daily Exercise

Remember, this routine is optional. Following the guidelines in chapters 8 through 11, check off the items that apply.

I performed my general warm-up and stretching routine at the proper RPE
____

I performed my pelvic stabilizer exercises in the order indicated ____

I performed my lower body exercises in the order indicated ____

I completed all my sets and reps ____ Amount of weight used ____

I performed my general warm-up at the proper RPE ____

I performed my specific warm-up at the proper RPE ____

I performed my energy system management exercises at the proper RPE
____

I performed my cooldown at the proper RPE ____

I stretched as needed ____

How I felt at the end of my workout _____

Day 7

Rest and Recovery Day

High-Performance Nutrition

Use the guidelines for high-performance nutrition in chapters 3 through 5. Also include what *time* you eat each meal.

Breakfast _____

Snack _____

Lunch _____

Snack _____

Dinner _____

Snack _____

Daily fluid intake _____
(Aim for ½ to 1 ounce per pound of body weight. Example: if you weigh 160 pounds, you should drink between one and a half and three 1.5 liter bottles of water.)

Coffee, tea, sodas _____
(Always drink these in moderation since they contain caffeine and sugar. Most of your daily fluid intake should be water.)

High-Performance Nutrition Supplementation

No supplementation.

No Exercise

Make this a true rest-and-recovery day. This practice will greatly enhance your body's energy and muscle-building capacity. See chapter 1 for the reasons behind taking rest-and-recovery days.

Resources

Medical Organizations

American Academy of Family Physicians
11400 Tomahawk Creek Parkway
Leawood, KS 66211-2672
www.familydoctor.org

American Heart Association (AHA)
National Center
7272 Greenville Avenue
Dallas, TX 75231
800-242-8721
www.americanheart.org

Centers for Disease Control and Prevention
National Center for Chronic Disease Prevention
   and Health Promotion
Division of Nutrition and Physical Activity
4770 Buford Highway NE
Atlanta, GA 303421
770-488-5820
www.cdc.gov/nccdphp/dnpa

National Cholesterol Education Program
NHLBI Health Information Center
P.O. Box 30105
Bethesda, MD 20824-0105
301-592-8573

National Mental Health Association
2001 North Beauregard Street, 12th Floor
Alexandria, VA 22311
800-969-NMHA
www.nmha.org

Nutrition

American Dietetic Association (ADA)
216 West Jackson Boulevard
Chicago, IL 60606-6995
800-877-1600; 312-899-0040; 312-899-4739 (FAX)
800-366-1655 (Consumer Hotline)
E-mails: hotline@eatright.org; infocenter@eatright
   .org

American Society for Clinical Nutrition (ASCN)
9650 Rockville Pike
Bethesda, MD 20814
301-530-7110; 301-571-1863 (FAX)
E-mail: secretar@acsn.faseb.org

The Glycemic Research Institute
601 Pennsylvania Avenue, NW, Suite 900
Washington, D.C. 20004
202-434-8270
www.glycemic.com; www.anndeweesallen.com

U.S. Food and Drug Administration
5600 Fishers Lane
Rockville, MD 20857-0001
888-463-6332
www.fda.gov

Fitness Organizations

American College of Sports Medicine (ACSM)
401 W. Michigan Street
Indianapolis, IN 46206-3233
317-637-9200
www.acsm.org

American Council on Exercise (ACE)
5820 Oberlin Drive, Suite 102
San Diego, CA 92121-3787
619-535-8227
www.acefitness.org

Cooper Institute for Aerobic Research (CIAR)
12330 Preston Road
Dallas, TX 75230
214-701-8001
www.cooperinst.org

The National Women's Health Information Center
8550 Arlington Boulevard, Suite 300
Fairfax, VA 22031
800-994-9662
800-220-5446 (TDD)
www.4woman.gov/fag/heartdise.htm

President's Council on Physical Fitness and Sports
Room 738-H Hubert H. Humphrey Building
200 Independence Avenue, SW
Washington, D.C. 20201-0004
www.fitness.gov

Shape Up America!
6707 Democracy Boulevard, Suite 306
Bethesda, MD 20817
301-493-5368
www.shapeup.org

Books

Anderson, Bob. *Stretching* (20th anniversary revised edition). Bolinas, CA: Shelter Publications, 2000.

————, Bill Pearl, Edmund R. Burke, and Jean Anderson. *Getting in Shape: 32 Workout Programs for Lifelong Fitness* (2nd edition). Bolinas, CA: Shelter Publications. 2002.

Brand-Miller, Janet, Thomas M. S. Wolever, and Kay Foster-Powell. *The Glucose Revolution: The Authoritative Guide to the Glycemic Index.* New York: Marlowe and Co., 1999.

Charnetski, Carl J., and Francis X. Brennan. *Feeling Good Is Good for You: How Pleasure Can Boost Your Immune System and Lengthen Your Life.* New York: Rodale Press, 2001.

Cowden, W. Lee, Ferre Akbarpour, Russ Dicarlo, and Burton Goldberg. *Longevity: Reverse the Aging Process and Stay Young with Clinically Proven Alternative Therapies.* Alternative Medicine.com, 2001.

Goglia, Philip L. *Turn Up the Heat: Unlock the Fat-Burning Power of Your Metabolism.* New York: Viking, 2002.

Murray, Michale T. *Dr. Murray's Total Body Tune-Up.* New York: Bantam, 2000.

Pearl, Bill. *Getting Stronger: Weight Training for Men and Women.* Bolinas, CA: Shelter Publications, 2000.

Shilstone, Mackie. *The Fat-Burning Bible: 28 Days of Foods, Supplements, and Workouts That Help You Lose Weight.* Hoboken, NJ: John Wiley & Sons, 2005.

————. *Lose Your Love Handles: A 3-Step Program to Streamline Your Waist in 30 Days.* New York: Perigee, 2001.

————. *Maximum Energy for Life: A 21-Day Strategic Plan to Feel Great, Reverse the Aging Process, and Optimize Your Health.* Hoboken, NJ: John Wiley & Sons, 2003.

Web Sites

www.eatright.org

Health Net
www.healthnet.com

Mackie Shilstone's Web site
www.mackieshilstone.com

Omerga Institute for Holistic Studies
www.omega-inst.org

Ochsner Health System
www.ochsner.org
www.myheartrisk.com
www.revivalsoy.com

Yoga Journal
www.yogajournal.com

*on*health
www.onhealth.com
www.coachu.com
www.WebMD.com

Index